THE TRANSFORMATIVE POWER OF METAPHOR IN THERAPY

Sana Loue, JD, PhD, MPH, MSSA, is a Professor in the School of Medicine of Case Western Reserve University in Cleveland, Ohio, and serves as the Director of the university's Center for Minority Public Health. She holds a BA in Social Welfare (University of West Florida), an MA in secondary education (University of West Florida), a degree in law (University of San Diego School of Law), an MPH degree with a concentration in epidemiology (San Diego State University), a PhD in epidemiology (University of California Los Angeles), a PhD in medical anthropology (Case Western Reserve University), and an MSSA degree with a concentration in mental health (Mandel School of Applied Social Sciences, Case Western Reserve University). She was ordained as an interfaith minister by The New Seminary. Prior to joining the faculty of Case Western Reserve University, Dr. Loue practiced immigration law and AIDS law for 14 years. Dr. Loue is the author of more than 70 peer-reviewed articles and more than 50 book chapters and has authored or edited more than 20 books. Her current research interests include the cultural context of HIV risk; HIV prevention interventions for marginalized populations including persons with severe mental illness and substance use disorders; family violence; research ethics; and forensic epidemiology.

The Transformative Power of Metaphor in Therapy

SANA LOUE,
JD, PhD, MPH, MSSA

SPRINGER PUBLISHING COMPANY

New York

Springer Publishing Company, LLC
11 West 42nd Street
New York, NY 10036
www.springerpub.com

Acquisitions Editor: Sheri W. Sussman
Production Editor: Rosanne Lugtu
Cover design: Joanne E. Honigman
Composition: Publication Services, Inc.

07 08 09 10/ 5 4 3 2 1

Library of Congress Cataloging-in-Publication Data

Loue, Sana.
    The transformative power of metaphor in therapy / Sana Loue.
       p.; cm.

    Includes bibliographical references.
    ISBN 978-0-8261-1952-0 (hardcover)
    1. Metaphor—Therapeutic use. I. Title.
    [DNLM: 1. Metaphor. 2. Psychotherapy—methods. 3. Self Concept. WM 420 L886t 2008]
    RC489.M47L68 2008
    616.89'14—dc22

                                                                    2008015044
Printed in the United States of America by Bang Printing.

Contents

A Note from the Author

This volume represents a compilation of moments in time in the lives of the individuals mentioned here, as they and I worked together to understand where they had been, who they were, and who and where they wished to be.

It is, as much, the story of my journey to that point in time where our travels met. My journey there has been both circuitous and purposeful, a tapestry of interwoven textures and colors of varied shades and depths.

My undergraduate education focused on social welfare. Although initially most interested in working with individuals, I quickly became disillusioned with the politics and bureaucracy that seemed to be an integral part of both a state agency and judicial system. This was the era of efforts to pass the Equal Rights Amendment, when judges and legislators and even civil servants could with impunity eject women out of their offices and chambers for having been so bold as to wear a pants suit.

Community organization suited both my then-temperament and my need for some visible product of my hours of work and effort. Not surprisingly, my disillusion increased in direct proportion to my encounters with unethical bureaucrats and self-serving politicians. My solution was law school.

I was fortunate to find my niche practicing immigration law and, in the later years during which I practiced, AIDS law. It fulfilled my need to work directly with people, to use the languages that I had studied, to learn about other cultures and other ways of being. In an effort to build a better foundation for the cases for which I was responsible, and to alleviate my sense that my world and/or I were becoming tunnel-visioned, I returned to graduate school to pursue a master's in public health degree.

The excitement of that experience propelled me to apply for admission to a PhD program in epidemiology. Here, I felt, I could integrate all of my interests and my desire to work directly with communities. I moved on to assume a faculty position at Case Western Reserve University, where I am now. As part of my PhD program, I had learned to design studies, to analyze quantitative data. I thought that would be the end of my formal education.

I was wrong. I needed more. It is an old saying that "the more you know, the more you don't know." Several years after I had assumed a faculty position, it became clear to me that I lacked both a theoretical foundation for examining the cultural context of illness risk and prevention and the skills for analyzing interview data (qualitative analysis). Because of the benefits offered to faculty and the caliber of our university, I was fortunate to be able to pursue a PhD in medical anthropology to acquire these skills.

Throughout these years, I continued to work with the same populations with which I had worked as an attorney—individuals who were poverty-stricken, non-English speakers, folks suffering from terminal diseases such as cancer and AIDS, individuals plagued with frightening hallucinations result-ing from their mental illness, men and women who had been tortured in their countries of origin by the military or the opposition or both. As an attorney, I represented many of those who were immigrants in deportation (now called removal) hearings, arguing against their removal from the United States. For those who were dying, I prepared living wills and powers of attorney.

As a faculty member, I continue to work with these same communities, but in a very different way. I am privileged to be welcomed into their commu-nities and homes, to hear from them what they need for better health.

It is through my work as a researcher with these very same marginal-ized communities that I came to realize a need to work with individuals and communities on yet a deeper level and expand further my under-standing of their world as seen through their lenses. I returned to graduate school yet again, to complete a master's degree in social work.

My field work afforded me the opportunity to continue to work with these same communities and individuals, in yet another dimension. Although numerous experiences in the context of my work as an attorney and a researcher provided fertile material for this volume, it was ultimately these field work experiences that provided the impetus to compose this volume, and those experiences continue as well to shape the direction of my research and my interactions with these communities.

I have had remarkable good fortune in my journey. I have studied and worked with amazingly brilliant people and have had the benefit of their experience. Still others have afforded me the privilege of their trust and have shared with me the most intimate of emotions and experiences as they struggled to make sense of their lives and the world around them. From each and every one of them, I have learned more about them, our intersecting realities, and myself. It is my hope that this volume provides you also with the opportunity to view their world and yours through yet another lens.

Acknowledgments

This book would never have been possible without the privilege of witnessing my clients in their journeys toward finding themselves. The individuals mentioned in this book represent clients with real problems and issues that they were addressing, although names, places, ages, and occupations have been changed or left ambiguous in order to protect their privacy. My co-participation in their journey has enabled me to learn a great deal about myself, about them, and about how to serve better as a witness and a guide in the therapeutic process.

Several people graciously reviewed preliminary drafts of some or all of these chapters and provided me with their insights. Foremost among them are Jerry Willing, LMSW, LMFT; Richard Romaniuk, PhD, LISW; and Victor Groza, PhD. Zane Jennings, MSW, LISW, deserves special thanks both for his careful reading and critique of these chapters and for his insights into my own process in working with metaphor. Both Zane Jennings and Kathi Overmeier-Gant are much appreciated for their openness and flexibility in the supervision that they provided to me during my field training in social work and my use of metaphors with clients in that context. A few clients also reviewed and commented on portions of this text, and although they wish to remain unnamed, they are also deserving of recognition. Sylvia Rimm, PhD, and Pierre Lehu provided me with the initial encouragement to move forward with the writing of this volume. Finally, I dedicate this book to Gussie Zand and Ruth Fogelman, who, through their own stories and storytelling, taught me the value of metaphor.

Introduction:

Peeking Through the Window: Why Use Metaphor?

Why, you might ask, is metaphor relevant to therapy and counseling?

As a skilled therapist, you know the need to have multiple approaches in your work with clients. What works for one client may not work for the next. You also know the difficulty of measuring change and growth; sometimes your client may "feel" that something is different from what it was when they first consulted with you, but may not be able to identify what that difference is.

Metaphor gives you another tool to use with clients. It is a way that both you and they can assess where they are, where they want to go with their therapy, and the distance that they travel in their therapeutic quest. And, as your clients gain insights from your use of metaphor with them, they can begin to understand the transformative power of metaphor and how it can help them in their journey even after they have left counseling. You can derive immense satisfaction at knowing that the lessons the client learned in counseling with you will continue to be useful to them.

The *American Heritage Dictionary of the English Language* (2000, p. 1104) defines the word *metaphor* as a "figure of speech in which a word or phrase that ordinarily designates one thing is used to designate another, thus making an implicit comparison" and "one thing conceived as representing another, a symbol." As an example, a river that winds its way through valleys and mountains and terminates at the ocean can be analogized to the course of one's life and the many difficulties and obstacles that one may encounter prior to attaining happiness, nirvana, or entry into God's Kingdom, depending upon one's beliefs.

Some metaphors can also be thought of as parables, short stories that teach a moral principle. Metaphors bear many similarities to parables and stories. All are ancient traditions that encourage creativity, connection with others, and the nurturance of dreams that may have not yet been spoken. Aesop's fables, for instance, are actually short stories that contain a moral lesson for the listener.

Many faith traditions impart their wisdom through the use of stories, parables, and metaphors. The Talmud, which dates back more than 2500 years, is a compendium of Jewish law and life that has been referred to as "an encyclopedia of Jewish life" (Bleefeld & Shook, 1998, p. 2). That portion of the Talmud known as the Aggadah contains parables, stories, and sermons that explain the law.

Christianity similarly relies on stories, parables, and metaphors. Much of Jesus's teachings were communicated through parable and metaphor (Stein, 1994), as illustrated by the following:

> I am the vine, you are the branches. Those who abide in me and I in them bear much fruit, because apart from me you can do nothing (John 15:5).
> I am the bread that came down from heaven (John 6:41).
> I am the bread that came down from heaven. If anyone eats of this bread, he will live forever. This bread is my flesh, which I will give for the life of the world (John 6:51).[1]

It has been said that Jesus's use of parables was effective as a teaching tool because he "used parables to present situations familiar to the rural poor" (Herzog, 1994, p. 27).

The metaphors referred to in this text have been derived from experience common to a wide range of individuals, and all are intended to stimulate thinking. Some may assist the client to identify and acknowledge different aspects of his or her personality. Others may be more suited to the task of examining relationships and interpersonal dynamics or of setting goals.

In the context of counseling, it is the client who fashions the story from the metaphor and who ultimately determines what, if any, lesson is to be learned from the story told. The use of metaphor rests on the assumption that, because illusions can never be destroyed directly (Kierkegaard, 1950), the best way to encourage and support change and growth is through story and parable (cf. Denning, 2005). Like the sugar that helps the medicine go down, the use of metaphor helps clients tolerate the unpleasantness that they may experience on their journeys to self-knowledge. A safe space is created in which the client can develop his or her own identity, sometimes embedded in story, using the metaphor as a basis. The metaphor creates the opportunity for the client as artist with palette in hand to paint a picture of himself or herself at

---

[1]Christians who believe in the Real Presence of Christ in the Eucharist, such as Catholics and Orthodox, consider John 6 to have a literal, not only a metaphorical, meaning.

a point in time or, as the writer, director, and producer of a play, to determine the beginning, middle, and hoped-for end of their drama. Maguire's observation regarding the importance of storytelling for children is equally relevant to the use of metaphor with adults:

> Storytelling gives children more scope for working out their dreamlike perceptions of life, for symbolically confronting its myriad opportunities and difficulties. It equips them with tools—images and words—that they can use to test their intuition and powers of judgment; and it safely and gently introduces topics that can later be discussed openly outside of the privileged world of storytelling (Maguire, 1985, p. 20).

Because the use of metaphor in counseling often leads to the client's formulation of a story, some readers may assume that the use of metaphor is narrative therapy by another name. Although metaphor can be used in conjunction with narrative therapy, these approaches are distinct. Like narrative therapy, the use of metaphor permits the client to externalize whatever may be thought of as "the problem" and to construct a story about part or all of his or her life. In the context of narrative therapy, the client may utilize metaphors to describe his or her problem or life; these metaphors originate with the client. In contrast, the use of metaphor as it is described in this text involves the counselor's identification of an object and an invitation to the client to utilize that object in describing his or her current situation or life.

This approach is advantageous in several respects. First, although the therapist may propose a particular metaphor to the client, whether and how the client chooses to use the metaphor remains entirely within the client's control. This encourages the therapist to work with the client from a position of neutrality. Second, the therapist's offer of new language in the form of metaphor serves as an indirect invitation to the client of change:

> Speaking isn't neutral or passive. Every time we speak, we bring forth reality. . . . What is important for psychotherapists is that change, whether it is change of belief, relationship, feeling, or self-concept, involves a change in language (Freedman & Combs, 1996, p. 29).

By offering metaphor, we give the client permission, opportunity, and a vehicle for potential change.

I used each of the 10 metaphors described in this volume with clients over a period of years during my supervised training in social work. (I mention here, again, my appreciation of the openness of my field advisors, Zane Jennings and Kathi Overmeier-Gant, to these ideas.) All of the clients described in this text had diagnoses of serious and persistent mental illnesses, including schizophrenia, bipolar disorder, major depression, and dysthymia. Some of these clients had been diagnosed with co-occurring substance use disorders, borderline personality disorder, and/or chronic physical conditions, such as diabetes, fibromyalgia, and irritable bowel syndrome. Clients ranged in age from 18 to their mid-70s and included men and women, those with insurance and those without, those who self-identified as white and those who self-identified as other than white, English speakers and non-English speakers, churchgoers and atheists, individuals of various sexual and gender identities and sexual orientations, those with employment and those without, folks with significant sources of emotional and/or financial support and those without either.

The use of metaphor in counseling has not, to the best of my knowledge, been tested empirically in a scientifically designed study. Nevertheless, it appears to be beneficial for some, both on an individual basis and in group work. Clients and students have come back years after their contact with me had ended to ask that I remind them of a particular metaphor and how it can be used, finding that it once again has the power to reveal to them hidden dimensions of their lives.

REFERENCES

American Heritage Dictionary of the English Language (4th ed.). (2000). Boston, MA: Houghton Mifflin Company.

Bleefeld, B. R., & Shook, R. L. (1998). *Saving the world entire and 100 other beloved parables from the Talmud.* New York: Penguin Putnam Inc.

Denning, S. (2005). *The leader's guide to storytelling: Mastering the art and discipline of business narrative.* San Francisco: Jossey-Bass.

Freedman, J., & Combs, G. (1996). *Narrative therapy: the social construction of preferred realities.* New York: W.W. Norton & Company.

Herzog, W. R. II. (1994). *Parables as subversive speech: Jesus as pedagogue of the oppressed.* Louisville, KY: Westminster/John Knox.

Kierkegaard, S. (1950). *The point of view.* London: Oxford University Press.

Maguire, J. (1985). *Creative storytelling: Choosing, inventing, and sharing tales for children.* New York: McGraw-Hill.

Stein, R. H. (1994). *The method and message of Jesus' teachings.* Louisville, KY: Westminster/John Knox.

SUGGESTIONS FOR FURTHER READING

Bandler, R., & Grinder, J. (1975). *The structure of magic I: A book about language and therapy.* Palo Alto, CA: Science and Behavior Books, Inc.

Bandler, R., & Grinder, J. (1976). *The structure of magic II.* Palo Alto, CA: Science and Behavior Books, Inc.

Collins, R., & Cooper, P. J. (1997). *The power of storytelling: Teaching through storytelling* (2nd ed.). Long Grove, IL: Waveland Press, Inc.

Zipes, J. (1995). *Creative storytelling: Building community, changing lives.* New York: Routledge.

THE TRANSFORMATIVE POWER OF
METAPHOR IN THERAPY

CHAPTER 1

Alphabet Soup:

Developing a Positive Self-Image

DEVELOPING SELF-ESTEEM

How do we know who we are? Our ideas about how we know ourselves derive from the work of William James, a nineteenth-century American psychologist. James distinguished between the I-self, which is the active observer and knower of experience, and the Me-self, or what is known about the self (James, 1892/1968). The I-self has also been referred to as the phenomenal self, and the Me-self as one's self-concept (Harter, 1988). Because the I-self is so difficult to perceive and assess, most research has focused on the development of the Me-self.

The term *self-concept* refers to individuals' knowledge of themselves, which can be thought of as the cognitive component of the self. This is to be distinguished from the concept of *self-esteem,* or what individuals feel about themselves; that is, the affective component of the self. The development of self-concept and self-esteem and the use of metaphor in working with individuals around these issues will be the focus of this chapter.

It is believed that our sense of ourselves results from our evaluation of the feedback that we receive from others (Cooley, 1902) and that we integrate the values and expectations of others in society into our sense of ourselves (Mead, 1934). This occurs through the cognitive processing of information that we receive. Individuals process information by organizing it into *schemas,* which are essentially frameworks that they use to understand the world around them and their own experiences; by adapting to new information through assimilating it into existing schemas or accommodating it through the modification of existing schemas or the construction of new ones; and by attempting to maintain cognitive balance, known as *equilibration* (Singer & Revenson, 1996). The concept of equilibration is similar to the biological concept of homeostasis, that is, maintaining a steady state. One's ability to know oneself depends on the maturation process of the brain and nervous system, which is genetically determined; one's experiences in the physical world; and interactions with other individuals (Markus & Nurius, 1986). Increasingly complex understandings of the self become possible with increasingly advanced cognitive development (Labouvie-Vief, Chiodo, Goguen, Diehl, & Orwoll, 1995).

Researchers have suggested that one's self-concept is stable and is very resistant to change once it has been formed. The stability of the self-concept has been explained as the result of a need to reduce ambiguity as quickly as possible (cognitive urgency) and to maintain cognitive closure (cognitive permanence) (Kruglanski & Webster, 1996). Information that is consistent with the existing schema may be more easily recognized and accepted, while information that is inconsistent is more likely to be ignored (Stangor & Ruble, 1989). Individuals who have developed a poor self-concept may consequently disregard all information that conflicts with their already-existing negative self-concept. For instance, individuals who think of themselves as failures because of the consistent negative feedback that they have received from others throughout their lives may be unable to perceive their own successes. Similarly, individuals with an unrealistically inflated self-concept may be reluctant or unwilling to hear that improvement may be possible and may react defensively to such suggestions.

As indicated, self-esteem can be thought of as the individual's feelings toward himself or herself, and as his or her self-evaluation along a negative-positive continuum. It is the evaluation that the I-self makes of the Me-self on a bad-good continuum. Individuals who have high self-esteem are those who are able to *realistically* evaluate themselves, accept and respect themselves, and decide that they have self-worth (Berk, 1991).

Self-esteem is believed to be "the most important requirement for effective behavior" (Coopersmith, 1967, p. 218). High self-esteem has been found to be associated with both good physical and good mental health (Antonucci and Jackson, 1983; Harter, 1988). Research has found that high self-esteem protects individuals from feelings of anxiety (Greenberg et al., 1992; Greenberg, Pyszczynski, Solomon, Pinel, Simon, & Jordan, 1993; Pyszczynsi, Greenberg, Solomon, Arndt, & Schimel, 2004) and motivates individuals to engage in behaviors that are self-protective and beneficial (Greenwald, 1988).

During childhood, individuals develop an assessment of themselves in disparate tasks, such as sports, making friends, or academic performance. During middle childhood, between the ages of 6 and 12, these disparate assessments are integrated into a synthesized self-assessment, or global self-esteem. Individuals' self-esteem is enlarged as they acquire new skills and participate in new experiences, which are then used as the basis for further self-assessments. To a great degree, individuals derive their self-esteem from the value that others attribute to them (Cooley, 1902), particularly from those who are significant figures in their lives, such as parents and other family members (Demo, Small, & Savin-Williams, 1987; Rosenberg, 1979; Ross & Broh, 2000; Schwalbe & Staples, 1991). Self-esteem can be thought of ultimately as the extent to which an individual's self-concept is consistent with his or her idealized self, in other words, with the way he or she would like to be (Atchley, 1982).

Many individuals with mental illness have both a poor self-concept and poor self-esteem, which then have an impact on their behavior. An examination of how mentally ill individuals are often perceived by others and the nature of the feedback that they receive from others is important to understanding why this might be the case.

Many individuals diagnosed with mental illness cease, in the minds of those who encounter them, to be individuals with a disease and become, instead, the disease and all that their label signifies. As an example, an individual with a diagnosis of schizophrenia may cease to be viewed by others as *an individual with schizophrenia* and becomes, instead, a *schizophrenic,* disaffirmed and diminished in importance.

As a result of this "mark," or stigma (Jones, Farina, Hastorf, Markus, Millar, & Scott, 1984), others may set the individual apart, may cease their "normal" conversations with him or her, and begin to isolate and marginalize him or her because of this mark (Laing, 1960, 1961; Launer, 1999). The "marked" individual may, as a consequence, experience feelings of rejection, loneliness, and depression (World Health Organization, 2001) and may redefine himself or herself in such a manner as to conform with the definition that is inherent in others' treatment of them or segregate himself or herself even further (Goffman, 1963; Scheff, 1984). One woman, diagnosed with bipolar disorder, wrote:

> Mental illness interacts with the way you define yourself from the instant it enters your life. There was a whole seventeen and a half years of living before this horrible episode descended upon me. Seventeen and a half years of wondering why I never felt quite right anywhere. Not in my home, not in my schools, not in my cliques, not with my boyfriends. Did this mental illness thing explain everything that ever happened to me? (Simon, 2002, p. 27)

Individuals may then behave in a way that they believe is consistent with others' treatment and expectations of them (Becker, 1963; Kitsuse, 1962; Link, Struening, Cullen, Shrout, & Dohrenwend, 1989; Scheff, 1984). They may act "crazy" or respond to situations in a manner that dooms them to further failure and/or rejection, perhaps even while unaware that they are doing so.

This is not to say that the development of and reliance on a diagnosis is ill-advised. Many benefits may come from the identification of an illness that is rooted in biology, including increased access to needed services, a broader array of beneficial therapeutic interventions, and the mobilization of family and community members to provide increased support (Carrey, 2007). However, all too often, the individual may adopt this "sick" identity as his or her own, together with the negative and threatening characteristics often attributed to such diagnoses: volatility, instability, incompetence, irresponsibility, violence, unpredictability. Not surprisingly, by the time individuals come into counseling, they have often assumed identities of failure and may be unable to point to any positive qualities that they may have. Other negative consequences may result, as well: an avoidance of help-seeking, nonadherence to prescribed medications, and the persistence of depressive symptoms (Chesney & Smith, 1999; Dinos, Stevens, Serfaty, Weich, & King, 2001; Goffman, 1963; Link, Struening, Neese-Todd, Asmussen, & Phelan, 2001; Link, Struening, Rahav, Phelan, & Nuttbrock, 1997; Roberts, 2005).

As seen, however, this self-identity as a sick person does not exist in a vacuum. Individuals do not conjure up such an image of themselves from nothing, but rather derive it as the result of interactions with those in their environment (Goffman, 1963; Scheff, 1984). First, the story that a client's family members tell about him or her cannot exist without support from the larger environment. Imbalances in the family dynamic, whether premised on age, sex, sexual orientation, color, earning power, or other factors, are supported by power imbalances in the larger culture (Reiss, 1985). Second, the story that clients then tell about themselves is directly a function of the story told about them by others and the story told to them about themselves by others. However unknowingly, they have co-constructed their own stories with individuals within and outside of their families. As one scholar noted, "[T]he story of my life is always embedded in the story of those communities from which I derive my identity . . . The possession of an historical identity and the possession of a social identity coincide. . . ." (MacIntyre, 1981, p. 221).

Some individuals may possess additional characteristics, such as their skin color or their sexual orientation, that "mark" them even further. In such instances, the intensity of their stigmatization and resulting marginalization may be compounded (Capitanio & Herek, 1999; Herek, 1999; Herek & Capitanio, 1999; Reidpath & Chan, 2005).

THE ALPHABET SOUP

Many times individuals who come into counseling are asked to relate their experiences and explain why they have chosen to seek counseling at that particular time. It is not uncommon for individuals with a chronic mental illness to report that they have sought help because of current or repeated difficulties at work or at home, or as a condition of probation. Frequently, their recitation of their experiences is devoid of any emotion or insight because it is a script that they have formulated, repeatedly verbalized, and perhaps even repeatedly acted out many times before. Their completion of formal intake forms may provide the professional with important information for insurance or program purposes, but it often fails to expand the client's self-evaluation skills.

I have used the metaphor of the alphabet soup as a mechanism to learn about both the client's life experiences and the client's self-concept and level of self-esteem. The client and I visualize together what it might feel like to be served a big bowl of alphabet soup. Most frequently, the client will describe the feeling of warmth that comes with the soup, not only of physical warmth, but also of emotional warmth, a sense of being cared for. Then I ask the client to imagine that every letter of the alphabet in that wonderful, warm soup signifies a positive quality that he or she has and invite the client to share a listing of these positive qualities with me.

To do this, I ask the client to list on a separate line of a sheet of notebook paper each letter of the alphabet and to choose a word for each letter that the client believes is a description of who he or she is. We then talk about each quality, what that quality signifies, how the client has used it in the past, and the meaning that the client ascribes to his or her use of it. Each experience that the client relates in conjunction with a particular adjective provides me with insight into significant events in the client's life, the client's strategies for responding to various situations, the client's perceptions of the significance of these events and the effectiveness of his or her responses to them, and the client's evaluation of himself or herself as an actor in relation to others.

This approach is less structured than a formal chronological life history, but it is often less threatening to clients. I have also found that because this strategy requires that clients tie their description of events to particular qualities that they own, they are provided with an enhanced opportunity for reflection and the development of an enhanced level of self-awareness. Their identification of positive qualities that they have used successfully can serve as a springboard for the improvement of their self-concept and the enhancement of their self-esteem from whatever level may exist at that time. The following case studies indicate how this metaphor can be used in working with clients.

USING THE STORY

Geoffrey (not his actual name), was 40 years old and struggling with the multiple "marks" of schizophrenia and homosexuality at the time of our first encounter. Geoffrey had been diagnosed two years previously with schizophrenia. Prior to the initial onset of illness symptoms, which included frightening auditory hallucinations, bouts of severe paranoia and anxiety, and a disabling inability to feel anything other than fear, he had been an instructor of adult education for many years and had been in a long-term relationship with his same-sex partner for almost two decades. Geoffrey had ended that relationship following the discovery of his partner's multiple instances of infidelity and his increased risk of exposure to HIV as a consequence of his partner's sexual behavior.

The progressive worsening of Geoffrey's illness resulted in his loss of employment, loss of income and medical insurance, and, ultimately, bankruptcy. Geoffrey had resided in a large urban area for most of his adult life, but, unable to support himself any longer, had moved in with his father and stepmother. They lived in a small, rural Midwestern community, known for its religious fundamentalism and conservative politics and often referred to by urban residents of the state as "dog and gun country." His father had "taken him in" out of a sense of responsibility to his son, but made clear that his son would not need medications if he were a "real" man and would get better if he would only "pull himself up by his bootstraps."

After a year with his father, Geoffrey relocated to a subsidized apartment. Although he had been faithfully following a prescribed medication regimen for several months at the time that we had this interaction, he continued to experience auditory hallucinations and bouts of severe paranoia and anxiety.

At this point, Geoffrey felt that his life, in his words, had been "a joke" and that he was a complete and utter failure. Each of the residents in the subsidized apartment building had been diagnosed with a severe mental illness; hence, he said, he was living in a "House of Dysfunction," providing yet another confirmation of his incompetence. Although he had self-identified as gay from an early age, he now felt that he should seek out Exodus, a group for homosexuals seeking to re-embrace heterosexuality. His schizophrenia, he believed, was a punishment from God for being gay, for this horrible being that he was at his core.

At the time of this initial encounter, Geoffrey had internalized homophobia. The term *homophobia* has been used to refer to antigay (including gay, lesbian, transgender, transsexual, and intersex) prejudice and discrimination that exists "out there," in the external world (Russell, 2007). In contrast, "internalized homophobia" is construed as that which resides within individuals. However, neither can exist without the other; one cannot internalize homophobia unless it first exists outside of oneself (Russell, 2007).

A task of primary importance was to help Geoffrey not only tell his story, but tell it in such a way that he could begin to recall the positive aspects of his life and his being, a process that White (2007) has referred to as the reauthoring of one's history. I used the metaphor of the alphabet soup with Geoffrey.

Geoffrey compiled a listing of his positive attributes. The use of the alphabet soup metaphor allowed Geoffrey to externalize the discussion and begin to examine his positive qualities without being required to accept ownership of them immediately, which he was unlikely to do in view of the negative identity conclusions that he had drawn from his life experiences and the diminished value placed on him by others. Geoffrey wrote:

Accepting	Nutty
Bleary-eyed	Observant
Compassionate	Perspicuous
Daring	Query
Ebullient	Realistic
Factual	Salubrious
Generous	Teacher
Heartfelt	Unaffected
Imaginative	Valiant
Jaunty	Wakeful
Kind	X-rated
Lasting	Youthful
Malleable	Zippy

I asked Geoffrey to explain how each of these adjectives applied to him and to give me an example of an event or occurrence in his life that reflected each quality that he had listed. We progressed through the words contained in Geoffrey's listing in an order that he chose, rather than alphabetically. This allowed Geoffrey greater control over the process and his level of vulnerability. As he focused on each adjective, I posed a series of questions to him in a manner designed to facilitate reflection and self-understanding. As an example, when Geoffrey talked about being "imaginative," I asked him to give me an example of a situation in which he was imaginative and to explain the circumstances that gave rise to that situation. He shared with me that he had been imaginative in how he had communicated ideas to his students so that they could more easily understand and integrate various concepts. I followed this discussion with questions such as:

- Does having been imaginative with your students tell you anything else about yourself?
- Are you ever imaginative now? In the same way or a different way?
- How did you know to do that?
- How did your students respond?

Similarly, when we came to the word *lasting*, Geoffrey described his friendship with a man that dated back to their initial meeting in grade school more than a quarter of a century earlier, and his efforts to maintain the friendship despite the many changes in each of their lives. I followed this disclosure with more "meaning questions" (Freedman & Combs, 1993), designed to understand the meaning and importance of the quality and its manifestation to Geoffrey:

- What does that say about yourself that you have been able to maintain this friendship over such a long period of time?
- Do you do this with all friendships? How do you decide which ones to be this committed to?
- Is this same quality noticeable in other parts of your life? In what way?
- Is there ever a time when it is not good to have this quality? In what situations?

As we progressed through Geoffrey's listing, he was gradually able to see his accomplishments, to take ownership of them, and to redefine himself as something other than a "failure," a "joke," or a "schizophrenic."

A number of the traits that Geoffrey listed reflected not only qualities that he perceived as positive, but also symptoms of Geoffrey's illness and its current impact. As such, the listing provided clues as to issues that could require attention in the context of our work together. For instance, Geoffrey had indicated that being "malleable" was a positive trait because it reflected flexibility and the ability to deal with even drastic changes in his life, even those over which he had no control. It also, though, reflected a trait that is often associated with schizophrenia: ambivalence or the inability to make a decision. Geoffrey was, indeed, flexible in his dealings with others, but he was also easily led into situations that could be potentially injurious to him, including anonymous sexual encounters.

Geoffrey's use of this word and his subsequent interpretation of the quality in his life allowed us to identify and explore the differences between situations that demand flexibility, those in which flexibility might be desirable but not required, and those in which flexibility might leave him vulnerable to abuse or betrayal. Geoffrey explained the need to be flexible in his definition of his responsibilities at work in order to contribute as a member of the team. He could be flexible in deciding which restaurant to go to for dinner with his friends. However, "flexibility" in the context of a new romantic-sexual relationship could be dangerous if it meant engaging in intercourse without a condom and thereby possibly exposing himself to HIV transmission.

Geoffrey still periodically struggles with feelings of low self-esteem and self-worth when he is confronted with events beyond his control. On most days, he is able to maintain a more balanced view of himself as a person and of his own accomplishments.

I also used the metaphor of the alphabet soup with Joseph, who initially had a difficult time identifying any positive qualities that he might have. He had met me through my activities with a minority young adult–focused community center, but he ultimately consulted me for counseling after he received a referral from another African American gay man with whom I had worked. Therapy, however, signified weakness. Joseph was deeply fearful that his carefully constructed, seemingly impenetrable veneer of defiance and toughness and his reputation for inflicting immediate retribution in response to any perceived affront would be irreparably diminished if others in the "'hood" learned that he was seeing a therapist, leaving him open to possible attack. His fear was, in large part, reality-based; three gay African American men in his community had been murdered at gunpoint during the six months preceding his initial consultation with me.

Despite his fears of the potential consequences if his therapy were to become known, Joseph began to see me because, as he said, he was "tired of feeling depressed." Joseph gradually and incrementally revealed the details of his life. He was one of four children, each of whom had a different father. His mother left him at a young age to be raised by his grandmother, and moved to a southern state, together with the other three children. His family constellation included, in addition to his grandmother, several male and female cousins, his mother's adult brother, an aunt, and, eventually, his grandmother's boyfriend. Although his grandmother had remained married, her husband, Joseph's grandfather, was rarely present and his whereabouts were usually unknown.

Joseph was raped by his uncle at the age of 9 or 10. Several years later, he was sexually abused by one of his older cousins. He expressed guilt because, unlike the episode with his uncle, he had enjoyed these sexual encounters with his cousin. These sexual activities somehow became known to the other members of his family, and Joseph was soon known as the "fag." When, as an adolescent, he visited his mother and other siblings down South, she accused him of sexually molesting his younger brother, which he has consistently denied doing. His mother responded to his denial by beating him with a pipe, resulting in injuries severe enough to his arm to require medical attention "for falling." He returned to live with his grandmother, who, he reported, increasingly insisted that he was "no good" and "all bad."

It was at this time, in 1999, that Joseph appeared to have suffered his first major depressive episode. The second occurred approximately 5 years later, following the break-up of his first long-term sexual-romantic relationship with another man of the same age. According to Joseph's description, his partner was abusive towards him even during the initial stages of the relationship. However, the combativeness became mutual over time, which Joseph attributed to his own efforts at self-defense against his partner's blows. Following this break-up, Joseph sought counseling through a publicly-funded program, but soon discontinued his sessions with the psychiatrist and the social worker, believing that the medications that he had been given were ineffective and that the psychiatrist was uninterested.

At the time Joseph consulted with me, he was in his early 20s and had not completed high school. He worked intermittently, often losing jobs because of absences and tardiness. He reported frequently bingeing on alcohol and periodically using marijuana. He continued to reside with his grandmother and her boyfriend, and had intermittent contact with his abusive uncle and cousin at family gatherings. He rarely communicated with his mother and siblings, with the exception of a younger brother who had moved in with one of his aunts who resided locally. His daily routine consisted of sleep until early afternoon, "hanging" with his friends, and drinking into the early hours of the following morning. Although he continued to be sexually impulsive, he reported deriving no pleasure from these anonymous sexual encounters and feeling "even more shitty" after each one. He described his life as purposeless and himself as a "loser" who had failed at everything and would never succeed at anything.

Initial assessment indicated that Joseph was suffering from dysthymia. He had lost interest in writing music, "hanging" with friends, and all other activities that he had previously found pleasurable. He alternated between periods of excessive sleep and insomnia. Although he had once been able to compose lyrics, some of which had been published, he reported that he was no longer "able to write feelings down" and "couldn't feel."

Joseph's alphabet soup, which encompassed most of the letters of the alphabet, consisted of the following:

Adventurous	Loyal
Brave	Meticulous
Control	Nice
Dynamic	Observant
Expressive	Practical
Friendly	Quick
Go-getter	Reliable
Honest	Sad
Intense	Talented
Joker	Understanding
Keyless	Vocal

Unlike the alphabet soup that Geoffrey had "cooked," which in many ways appeared to accurately reflect the positive aspects of his personality and his interactions with others, Joseph's listing of his positive qualities suggested that he was unable to distinguish between those that were aspirational or idealized and those that he actually possessed. For instance, although he characterized himself as reliable, he had forgotten numerous scheduled meetings with his record agent, to the point that his agent dropped him from his list of clients. This behavior was not confined to interactions with his agent but also characterized his dealings with his grandmother, his uncle, his instructors at school, and his employers.

I did not raise Joseph's lack of reliability with him directly. If I had done so, he would likely have terminated counseling because of the still tenuous state of our therapeutic relationship and the ensuing feeling of danger and vulnerability. Instead, I repeatedly returned to his self-description with more questions that sought to help Joseph both question his reality and discover his own answers: Can you describe a situation in which you were reliable? What helped you to be reliable then? How important is it for you to be like that? Why? Joseph gradually came to realize that there were situations in which he was reliable and those in which he was not.

Because Joseph already had an image of himself as a "loser," it was important that this self-realization not become the focus of self-blame and result in a further diminution of Joseph's self-worth. As Joseph came to realize how frequently he had been unreliable, we identified and increasingly emphasized in our work together those circumstances and factors that seemed to encourage and support him in being reliable. This process provoked additional questions for Joseph: How can you bring these factors into your life more often? How can you emphasize them more so that they can help you to be reliable?

Joseph's process of listing his self-perceived positive attributes led to an awareness of the need to develop a realistic self-appraisal that encompassed the strengths that Joseph possessed and the behaviors that required change if he were to succeed in his creative ventures and interpersonal relations. Over time, as we progressively addressed each of the enumerated qualities in the context of actual situations, Joseph came to realize that he had painted an idealized picture of himself and indicated that he may have done this as a mechanism to ward off feelings about his own incompetence. The questions that I had posed to Joseph were critical to the development of this insight; indeed, "[e]very time we ask a question, we're generating a possible version of a life" (D. Epston, quoted in Cowley & Springen, 1995, p. 74). One day, he exclaimed in amazement and with laughter, "You read me all along!" meaning that I had recognized from the beginning that what he had said about himself with the listing had not been entirely accurate.

Charonda, a 35-year-old African American woman, had been diagnosed with bipolar disorder. When I first met her, she had recently been discharged from the hospital and had entered an intensive outpatient treatment program that utilized cognitive behavioral therapy. I was provided with only Charonda's diagnosis and details of her hospitalization and medication regimen. Our use of the alphabet soup both afforded Charonda an opportunity for self-reflection and self-assessment and provided me with basic information about her current living situation.

Charonda's list and accompanying explanations of her qualities reflected not only her perceptions of herself, but also what she believed others thought of her.

Active	I do love to stay active.
Believer	I believe in the future and my family.
Caring	I care about everyone.
Daughter	(Good). All the way there for my mother.
Enjoy	People say that I'm a joy to be around.
Friendly	Everyone should be this way.
Giving	I give to everyone if possible.
Helpful	Love to give in the time of need
Intelligent	Knowledgeable about many things
Joyful	Always happy to be around
Kind	Never too mean
Loving	Love is the best of all. I just about love everything.
Mother	(Good). 3 great kids, single mother
Neat	Always cleaning
Original	I love myself. My mom says I'm deep.
Pretty	I think I'm pretty.
Quick	Get the job done quickly
Respectful	Respect others
Successful	I'm happy.
Talk	Love to meet people
Useful	Have a way to use things in another way
Vibrant	Always smiling
Worker	Boss says I'm a good worker.
X-ray	Kids say I see all things.
Young-at-heart	35 and still going on, love to walk, play, run, etc.
Zoo	I love the zoo & the cats & fish.

Charonda reported that this was a difficult exercise for her and that she had to struggle to identify good qualities about herself. Her listing and explanations give us clues as to what issues might arise during her efforts to heal and to move forward with her life. Consider, for instance, the following:

I care about everyone.

All the way there for my mother.

Everyone *should* be this [Friendly] way.

Always happy to be around

Always smiling

While not conclusive, Charonda's frequent nonuse of "I" in describing her own qualities suggested that she may have difficulty acknowledging herself. In addition, her phrasing suggests that Charonda may view situations in absolute terms (*should, always*) and that there may be boundary issues with others (*everyone, all the way there*).

Charonda and I used the self-descriptions contained in her list as a springboard to discuss the meaning of love and what it meant to Charonda to think of herself and to be thought of by others as "giving," "caring," "helpful," "loving," and "useful." We explored the variety of responses that Charonda had received to her efforts at being helpful and loving, and how these responses had affected her life. Gradually, Charonda was able to identify situations in which she had neglected herself in the process of helping others and had felt drained as a result. Charonda's apparent altruism was actually a "pseudo-altruism," masking her lack of self-acceptance and providing a mechanism for self-destructiveness (see Seelig & Rosof, 2001).

I have also used this exercise in a group setting with individuals with diagnoses of bipolar disorder and major depression. I find the use of the alphabet soup metaphor particularly helpful when starting a new group because it serves as a relatively nonthreatening invitation to people who do not know each other to share who they are. It also provides an opportunity for me to understand on a preliminary basis how each individual in the group perceives himself or herself, the context of that perception, and how they choose to relate to others who are new to them.

To begin, I provide pencil and paper to the group participants and invite them to list one of their qualities for each letter of the alphabet. I have found it helpful to provide pencils rather than pens to emphasize to participants that they can feel free to change their responses and so that they are less likely to become preoccupied with the neatness or sloppiness of their paper.

After everyone has written down their list of alphabetical qualities, individuals take turns reading their lists out loud. They are each given an opportunity to choose one quality that they mentioned and explain in greater detail when and how they use it. After each individual has read his or her list and explained no more than one quality, other members of the group have the opportunity to comment on the list that has been read, indicating which of the qualities they have observed and which of the qualities identified by the person about himself or herself may have been helpful to other members of the group. Many individuals do not have an awareness of how they manifest their qualities through their interactions with others and how those interactions impact others. This exchange provides valuable feedback to group participants.

In other instances, group members may be unable to identify their own positive traits or may be reluctant to do so. The reading of their incomplete lists to other members of the group provides an opportunity to consider the observations of other group members and to decide whether the qualities that they experience from an individual are to be owned as their own. Marsha and Susan, both participants in an intensive outpatient program for individuals with bipolar disorder, completed only portions of their alphabet. Their lists are placed side by side here to demonstrate both the diversity and the similarity of responses that can arise in the group context. Contributions from other group participants to their lists are placed in brackets. "Missing" is indicated in brackets for those letters for which the individual could not think of a trait or characteristic.

MARSHA	SUSAN
Act politely	Assertive
Believe in God	[Believer]
Compassionate	Caring
Do nice things for others	Daring
Empathy for others	[Enjoying]
Forgiving	Fighter
G [missing]	Giving
Helpful	Humorous
Include others	Intelligent
J [missing]	Jokes around
Kind	Kind
Listen	Loving
Minister to others	Mindful
Nice	Nice
[Open]	Original
Pure thoughts	Patient
[Quality]	Quiet
R [missing]	Realistic
Smile	Silent

Talk	Timely
Uphold people	Unique
V [missing]	Vivacious
W [missing]	Weird

There are significant differences in the listings prepared by Susan and Marsha. Marsha explains herself almost entirely in relation to others: Do nice things for others, Empathy for others, Forgiving, Helpful, Include others, Minister to others, Uphold people. Although Marsha may actually relate to others in this manner, this listing reflects what she does. The listing necessarily prompts the question: Who is Marsha apart from her actions? This suggests issues that, over time, Marsha herself may wish to address and, in fact, may need to address if she is to receive the support that she needs from others in her life to deal effectively with her mental illness.

The use of the alphabet soup metaphor in group is not without its dangers. Sometimes, an individual may want to disclose details of a situation that the group is not ready to hear because of the nature of the issues involved, the focus of the particular group, or the stage of the group's development. An individual may later regret, be embarrassed by, or be harmed by a very personal disclosure that he or she impulsively makes. Because the use of this metaphor encourages clients to self-disclose, the therapist must be mindful of the nature, depth, and timing of the disclosures that are made in the group context and be prepared to intercede to inhibit or restrain self-disclosures that may be self-harmful in this context.

As an example, disclosure by Geoffrey of his homosexuality to group co-participants residing with him in his "House of Dysfunction" would likely have resulted in ostracism from the group, potential harassment, and even possible violence in view of the extremism of members' religious beliefs and the homophobia that prevailed in the larger community in which he lived. Accordingly, I will not use the alphabet soup metaphor in a group setting if I have reason to believe or sense at the beginning of the group session that a participant may be prone to naïve and/or self-destructive disclosures or that I might have difficulty modulating the group rhythm and dynamic.

REFERENCES

Antonucci, T. C., & Jackson, J. (1983). Physical health and self-esteem. *Family and Community Health, 6,* 1–9.

Atchley, R. (1982). The aging self. *Psychotherapy: Theory, Research, and Practice, 19,* 388–396.

Becker, H. S. (1963). *Outsiders: Studies in the sociology of deviance.* New York: Free Press.

Berk, L. (1991). *Child development* (2nd ed.). Boston: Allyn & Bacon.

Capitanio, J. P., & Herek, G. M. (1999). AIDS-related stigma and attitudes toward injecting drug users among black and white Americans. *American Behavioral Scientist, 42(7),* 1148–1161.

Carrey, N. (2007). Practicing psychiatry through a narrative lens: Working with children, youth, and families. In C. Brown & T. Augusta-Scott (Eds.), *Narrative therapy: Making meaning, making lives* (pp. 77–101). Thousand Oaks, California: Sage Publications.

Chesney, M. A., & Smith, A. W. (1999). Critical delays in HIV testing and care: The potential role of stigma. *American Behavioral Scientist, 42,* 1162–1174.

Cooley, C. (1902). *Human nature and the social order.* New York: Scribner.

Coopersmith, S. (1967). *The antecedents of self-esteem.* San Francisco, California: Freeman.

Cowley, G., & Springen, K. (1995). Rewriting life stories. *Newsweek,* April 17, 70–74.

Demo, D. H., Small, S. A., & Savin-Williams, R. C. (1987). Family relations and the self-esteem of adolescents and their parents. *Journal of Marriage and the Family, 49,* 705–715.

Dinos, S., Stevens, S., Serfaty, M., Weich, S., & King, M. (2001). Stigma: The feelings and experiences of 46 people with mental illness. *British Journal of Psychiatry, 184,* 178–191.

Freedman, J., & Combs, G. (1993). Invitations to new stories: Using questions to explore alternative possibilities. In S. Gilligan & R. Price (Eds.), *Therapeutic conversations* (pp. 291–303). New York: W. W. Norton & Company.

Goffman, E. (1963). *Stigma: Notes on the management of spoiled identity.* New York: Touchstone.

Greenberg, J., Pyszczynski, T., Solomon, S., Pinel, E., Simon, L., & Jordan, K. (1993). Effects of self-esteem on vulnerability-denying defensive distortions: Further evidence of an anxiety-buffering function of self-esteem. *Journal of Experimental Social Psychology, 29,* 229–231.

Greenberg, J., Solomon, S., Pyszczynski, T., Rosenblatt, A., Burling, J., Lyon, D., et al. (1992). Why do people need self-esteem? Converging evidence that self-esteem serves as an anxiety-buffering function. *Journal of Personality and Social Psychology, 63,* 913–922.

Greenwald, A. (1988). A social-cognitive account of the self's development. In D. K. Lapsley & F. C. Powers (Eds.), *Self, ego, and identity: Integrative approaches* (pp. 30–42). New York: Springer-Verlag.

Harter, S. (1988). The construction and conversation of the self: James and Cooley revisited. In D. K. Lapsley & F. C. Power (Eds.), *Self, ego, and identity: Integrative approaches* (pp. 43–70). New York: Springer-Verlag.

Herek, G. M. (1999). AIDS and stigma. *American Behavioral Scientist, 42*(7), 1106–1116.

Herek, G. M., & Capitanio, J. P. (1999). AIDS stigma and sexual prejudice. *American Behavioral Scientist, 42*(7), 1130–1147.

James, W. (1968). In C. Gordon & K. J. Gergen (Eds.), *The self in social interaction.* New York: Wiley. (Adapted from *Psychology,* by W. James, 1892, New York: Henry Holt.)

Jones, E. E., Farina, A., Hastorf, A., Markus, H., Millar, D. S., & Scott, R. A. (1984). *Social stigma: The psychology of marked relationships.* New York: W. H. Freeman.

Kitsuse, J. L. (1962). Societal reaction to deviant behavior: Problems of theory and method. *Social Problems, 9,* 247–256.

Kruglanski, A. W., & Webster, D. M. (1996). Motivated closing of the mind: "Seizing" and "freezing." *Psychological Review, 103*(2), 263–283.

Labouvie-Vief, G., Chiodo, L. M., Goguen, L. A., Diehl, M., & Orwoll, L. (1995). Representations of self across the life span. *Psychology and Aging, 10*(3), 404–415.

Laing, R. D. (1960). *The divided self: An existential study in sanity and madness.* Harmondsworth, U.K.: Penguin.

Laing, R. D. (1961). *Self and others.* Harmondsworth, U.K.: Penguin.

Launer, J. (1999). A narrative approach to mental health in general practice. *British Medical Journal, 318,* 117–119.

Link, B. G., Struening, E. L., Cullen, F. T., Shrout, P. E., & Dohrenwend, B. P. (1989). A modified labeling theory approach to mental disorders: An empirical assessment. *American Sociological Review, 54*(3), 400–423.

Link, B. G., Struening, E. L., Neese-Todd, S., Asmussen, S., & Phelan, J. C. (2001). The consequences of stigma for the self-esteem of people with mental illness. *Psychiatric Services, 52*(12), 1621–1626.

Link, B. G., Struening, E. L., Rahav, M., Phelan, J. C., & Nuttbrock, L. (1997). On stigma and its consequences: Evidence from a longitudinal study of men with dual diagnoses of mental illness and substance abuse. *Journal of Health and Social Behavior, 38,* 177–190.

MacIntyre, A. (1981). *After virtue: A study in moral theory.* London: Duckworth.

Markus, H., & Nurius, P. (1986). Possible selves. *American Psychologist, 41,* 954–969.

Mead, G. H. (1934). *Mind, self, and society.* Chicago: University of Chicago Press.

Pyszczynski, T., Greenberg, J., Solomon, S., Arndt, J., & Schimel, J. (2004). Why do people need self-esteem? A theoretical and empirical review. *Psychological Bulletin, 130,* 435–468.

Reidpath, D. D., Chan, K. Y. (2005). A method for the quantitative analysis of the layering of HIV-related stigma. *AIDS Care, 17*(4), 425–432.

Reiss, D. (1985). Commentary: The social construction of reality—The passion within us all. *Family Process, 24,* 254–257.

Roberts, K. J. (2005). Barriers to antiretroviral medication adherence in young HIV-infected children. *Youth & Society, 37(2),* 230–245.

Rosenberg, M. (1979). *Conceiving the self.* New York: Basic Books.

Ross, C. E., & Broh, B. A. (2000). The roles of self-esteem and the sense of personal control in the academic achievement process. *Sociology of Education, 73,* 270–284.

Russell, G. M. (2007). Internalized homophobia: Lessons from the Mobius strip. In C. Brown & T. Augusta-Scott (Eds.), *Narrative therapy: Making meaning, making lives* (pp. 151–173). Thousand Oaks, California: Sage Publications.

Scheff, T. J. (1984). *Being mentally ill: A sociological theory* (2nd ed.). New York: Aldine de Gruyter.

Schwalbe, M. L., & Staples, C. L. (1991). Gender differences in sources of self-esteem. *Psychology Quarterly, 54,* 158–168.

Seelig, B. J., & Rosof, S. R. (2001). Normal and pathologic altruism. *Journal of the American Psychoanalytic Association, 49(3),* 933–959.

Simon, L. (2002). *Detour: My bipolar road trip in 4-D.* New York: Atria Books.

Singer, D. G., & Revenson, T. A. (1996). *A Piaget primer: How a child thinks* (rev. ed.). New York: Penguin Books.

Stangor, C., & Ruble, D. N. (1989). Strength of expectancies and memory for social information: What we remember depends on how much we know. *Journal of Experimental Social Psychology, 25,* 18–35.

White, M. (2007). *Maps of narrative practice.* New York: W. W. Norton & Company.

World Health Organization. (2001). *Mental health problems: The undefined and hidden burden.* (Fact Sheet No. 218). Retrieved August 8, 2007, from http://www.who.int/mediacentre/factsheets/fs218/eng/print.html

SUGGESTIONS FOR FURTHER READING

Same-Sex Relationships

Greenan, D.E. & Tunnell, G. (2003). *Couple therapy with gay men.* New York: Guilford Press.

Island, D., & Letellier, P. (1994). *Men who beat the men who love them: Battered gay men and domestic violence.* New York: Harrington Park Press.

Schizophrenia

Nasar, S. (1998). *A beautiful mind.* New York: Touchstone.

Pantelis, C., Nelson, H. E., & Barnes, T. R. E. (Eds.). (1996). *Schizophrenia: A neuropsychological perspective.* West Sussex, England: John Wiley & Sons Ltd.

Sexual Orientation

Cohler, B. J., & Galatzer-Levy, R. M. (2000). *The course of gay and lesbian lives: Social and psychoanalytic perspectives.* Chicago: University of Chicago Press.

Garnets, L. D., & Kimmel, D. C. (Eds.). *Psychological perspectives on lesbian, gay, and bisexual experiences.* (2nd ed.). New York: Columbia University Press.

CHAPTER 2

The Bicycle:

*How to Learn from the Past and
Move Toward the Future*

DEVELOPING A FUTURE ORIENTATION AND
PROBLEM-SOLVING SKILLS

Shakespeare tells us in his play *As You Like It* that there are seven distinct
stages of our lives, each characterized by specific life circumstances:

All the world's a stage,
And all the men and women merely players:
They have their exits and their entrances;
And one man in his time plays many parts,
His act being seven ages. At first the infant,
Mewling and puking in the nurse's arms.
And then the whining school-boy, with his satchel
And shining morning face, creeping like snail
Unwillingly to school. And then the lover,
Sighing like furnace, with a woeful ballad
Made to his mistress' eyebrow. Then a soldier,
Full of strange oaths and bearded like the pard,
Jealous in honour, sudden and quick in quarrel,
Seeking the bubble reputation
Even in the cannon's mouth. And then the justice,
In fair round belly with good capon lined,
With eyes severe and beard of formal cut,
Full of wise saws and modern instances;
And so he plays his part. The sixth age shifts
Into the lean and slipper'd pantaloon,
With spectacles on nose and such on side,
His youthful hose, well saved, a world too wide

Portions of this chapter were previously published in *Health Issues Confronting Minority Men Who Have Sex with Men*
(© Springer Science + Business Media, LLC, 2008).

21

For his shrunk shank; and his big manly voice,
Turning again toward childish treble, pipes
And whistles in his sound. Last scene of all,
That ends this strange eventful history,
Is second childishness and mere oblivion,
Sans teeth, sans eyes, sans taste, sans every thing.

As You Like It, act II, Scene 7, 139

Shakespeare's musings about the various stages of our lives are remarkably similar to the model of development that was formulated by Erik Erikson. Erikson theorized that individuals develop and progress through distinct stages of growth over the life course, each characterized by specific tasks that must be learned in order to acquire the skills necessary to navigate successfully through life's many and varied demands and to progress to the next stage of development. These stages include four preadolescent stages, adolescence (teenage years), early adulthood (20s and 30s), middle-age (40s and 50s), and later life (age 60 and older) (Erikson, 1964, 1968, 1997). Although the stages of development are presumed to be universal, individuals may differ in how they navigate these phases, as a result of variations in personality, culture, life events, and general circumstances.

The development of a future orientation and goal-setting are critical tasks of adolescence. Enhancement of these skills may decrease adolescents' risk of engaging in health-compromising behaviors (Perry & Jessor, 1985), such as substance use, and facilitate their healthful development. For instance, among adolescents, having concrete and realistic goals has been found to be associated with better academic performance (Gaa, 1979; Miller & Kelley, 1994; Trammel & Schloss, 1994).

The accomplishment of one's goals requires the development of problem-solving skills. Among adolescents, the development of these skills has been linked to reduced levels of anxiety, a better self-concept, the formation of an internal locus of control, and improved study habits and academic performance (Elliott, Godshell, Shrout, & Witty, 1990; Hay, Byrne, & Butler, 2000; Heppner, Reeder, & Larson, 1983; Nigro, 1996).

Individuals with a severe mental illness may experience difficulties in developing a future orientation and problem-solving skills. Depending on the particular mental illness, this may be associated with an inability to concentrate, indecisiveness, insecurity, difficulty handling stress or conflict, or the loss of paper and people skills (*DSM-IV-TR,* 2000; cf. Berger & Berger, 1991; Irwin, 1998).

The development of a future orientation may be particularly difficult for individuals who have experienced severe trauma. Bessel van der Kolk, a preeminent scholar in the field of trauma, observed (1996b, p. 204), "If it is true that traumatized people tend to become fixated at the emotional and cognitive level at which they were traumatized . . . they will tend to use the same means to deal with contemporary stresses that they used at the stage of development at which the trauma first occurred."

A number of theories have been advanced in an attempt to understand why some individuals are unable to move past the traumatic experiences. Research has demonstrated that trauma affects people on multiple levels of *biological* functioning (van der Kolk, 1996a). Studies suggest that individuals with posttraumatic stress disorder may have abnormalities in their limbic systems (Bremner et al., 1995; Saxe, Vasile, Hill, Bloomingdale, & van der Kolk, 1992), which may impact the manner in which emotionally charged memories are processed. For instance, the amygdala, one of the components of the limbic system, is responsible for the conditioning of fear responses, the attachment of affect to neural stimuli, and the establishment of associations between sensory modalities. A lesion in this area of the brain may result in a loss of fear responses and of meaningful social interaction (van der Kolk, 1996a). The hippocampus, another component of this system, is responsible for recording in memory the temporal and spatial dimensions of experience. It is particularly important in short-term memory; information is held in short-term memory and then is either immediately forgotten or processed as a more permanent memory. The ability to learn from experience depends, in part, on whether the short-term memory process functions adequately (van der Kolk, 1996a).

I once read, "You can only move as fast as the slowest part of you is able to move." If we consider Erikson's framework, we can envision through a variety of scenarios how this might occur as individuals pass through successive stages of life. Some individuals acquire the skills necessary to pass successfully from one stage to the next, processing and incorporating what they can learn from their environment and their experiences and carrying these lessons with them as they look and move forward in life. Others may remain "stuck" or "frozen," unable to integrate their experience(s) and move forward developmentally, although they continue to age chronologically. Still others may move forward developmentally in some aspects but not in others, so it is as if they are moving to their future while part of them remains rooted to the past. These various scenarios invite the use of the bicycle as a metaphor.

THE STORY OF THE BICYCLE

Think of riding a bicycle. Maybe you are envisioning a ride on a mountain bike down a winding path through a green, wooded, peaceful forest. Or perhaps you are on a 12-speed racing through traffic in a large city. Still others of you may be charging forward on a roaring motorcycle, winding around mountainous curves on a highway that hugs the ocean coast.

Whatever your image, you must be aware of what it is that you are passing and where you have been, all the while looking forward to see where you are going. An unremitting gaze towards your past route instead of the approaching path may land you against a tree, in a ditch or, worse yet, on a fatal collision course.

And so it is with life. It is important to know where we have been; to learn from our past and honor the experiences that we have had, which may range from the joyous to the torturous; to see mindfully where we are at the present; and to look toward our path into the future. If we live in the past while trying to move toward the future, we are unlikely to make much progress beyond where we were when we actually lived in the past.

We can see how this metaphor worked for Joseph, whom you may remember from his work with the alphabet soup, described in the first chapter. Joseph's family was, by all standards, quite poor. Joseph's grandmother supported them using her social security checks and food stamps. There was no household budget; food, rent, and lights depended on receipt of the expected check. Bills were paid in cash, in person, on the day that they were due, or maybe several days past the due date. Economic survival was tenuous at best, and there was no planning past the next day.

Joseph lamented this situation because he felt as though he would never achieve what he called a "good life" and a "meaningful life" if he were constantly living such an unstable existence. When asked what he could learn as he "rode" past this on his metaphorical bicycle, he quickly responded that he needed to plan better for his financial future, but did not know how to do this. We talked about what it means to have a budget and to live within one's budget.

At the next session, Joseph presented me with what he called his "Independence Budget." He listed his monthly income and his anticipated expenses each month, which included rent, utilities, a car note, gas, groceries, and entertainment. He set aside 15% of his monthly income to put into savings to cover upcoming anticipated expenses, such as car maintenance costs, and any unanticipated expenses that might arise. He had also applied for a credit card with a low credit limit and considered charging a few expenses each month and paying the bill immediately when due, in an effort to establish credit for himself. The establishment of a good credit history, he indicated, would be a necessity if he were to ever be able to purchase his own home. He had learned from his past, was cognizant of his present circumstances, and was looking toward the future, lessons in hand.

You may also recall Geoffrey's circumstances from the work that he did with the alphabet soup. Because of the symptoms of schizophrenia that he suffered,

Geoffrey had lost his job, his health insurance, and his home, and ultimately filed for bankruptcy. He was deeply embarrassed about his inability to have paid his bills and the consequent bankruptcy. We used the bicycle metaphor to explore what he had learned from this experience. Geoffrey concluded that, although he had been able to save some money prior to the onset of his illness, he had not developed a regular plan of saving for contingencies and had been too eager to spend money that he had not yet earned by using credit cards for purchases. He resolved not to buy most things for which he did not have the cash. Towards the end of the seven years following his bankruptcy, Geoffrey was able to secure an auto loan for a new car and regularly made payments in order to rehabilitate his credit rating. Rather than allowing himself to be drowned in feelings of embarrassment and shame because of the bankruptcy and the illness that helped to bring it about, Geoffrey used this past experience to learn about the importance of planning and saving. He could then use this knowledge to move toward the future, building a solid road as he did so.

Margaret's situation, however, illustrates what can happen when someone continues to focus only on what he or she has already passed on the metaphorical bicycle, rather than learning from it and focusing on their present route and what lies ahead. When I met Margaret, she was in her mid-40s and married to an engineer. They had one child in his mid-20s, who was unemployed and living at home with them. Margaret had been trained in an ancillary health field, but she had ceased working over a decade previously because of the increasing severity of her bipolar disorder. Margaret's efforts at returning to work during intermittent periods of relative mental stability were generally short-lived. Each attempt was interrupted by the occurrence of what Margaret characterized as unexpected and insurmountable obstacles: chronic body aches, difficulty driving because of inclement weather, another self-constructed crisis befalling their son.

Although Margaret had been in therapy with her psychologist and on a medication regimen for her bipolar disorder for over a decade, she continued to focus her attention and her energy on her experiences during her prepubescent and adolescent years. She had little or nothing to say of her life in the present and was unable to formulate plans or a vision for her future. Margaret's complaints about her past were those that many individuals have of their parents as they are growing up: that another sibling was the parental favorite, that a parent wouldn't purchase something that the child wanted, and that one or another sibling "had it easier." When Margaret spoke of these events, it was as if she were still living them, rather than remembering them. In fact, she had not changed her style of dress, her hairstyle, or her style of makeup in over two decades, so her appearance, in addition to the content of her speech, gave the impression that she was, indeed, living in a past era.

However, Margaret avoided speaking about the violence that she had witnessed as a child, which I learned about from others who knew her history. Her parents had divorced when she was in her late 20s. Their relationship had been volatile, rocky, and sometimes so brutal that she had feared that her mother would be killed. Her mother suffered from severe and chronic depression. Her father, who as a child had been severely abused physically by an alcoholic father and whose cognitive abilities and level of self-awareness were at a relatively low level, railed against the world for the injustices that had fallen upon him, believing himself to be the second coming of Job, the Biblical figure whose faith in God was tested by his immeasurable suffering, brought upon him as the result of a wager between God and Satan.

Margaret had attempted suicide on several occasions and had been hospitalized following each attempt. Although one psychiatrist had diagnosed her with co-occurring alcoholism, both she and one of her psychologists rejected this diagnosis; in her mind, the rejection signified permission to continue to drink.

What became increasingly clear over time was that Margaret responded to individuals whom she perceived as threatening or who reminded her in some way of a parent as if they were actually her parents. She assumed the demeanor of an accusing victim, as if the individuals with whom she was interacting had committed an unidentified and unidentifiable wrong against her that demanded rectification and retribution. The cause of all conflicts, whether at work with coworkers or supervisors or at home with her husband or son, was attributed to the other party, much as a child with his hand in the cookie jar blames someone else for the missing cookies. Even in her mid-40s, Margaret perpetuated with others the drama that she and her parents had scripted, unable to go beyond this past route to form healthier and more mature relationships.

In addition to having bipolar disorder, Margaret was experiencing what has been referred to as a "disorder of extreme stress not otherwise specified (DESNOS)" (van der Kolk, 1996b). Unlike the recognized diagnosis of posttraumatic stress disorder, which encompasses symptoms resulting from a single, identifiable traumatic event (*Diagnostic and Statistical Manual of Mental Disorders,* revised 4th ed.; *DSM-IV-TR*; American Psychiatric Association, 2000), DESNOS is a proposed diagnostic category for the psychological injury that may result from ongoing exposure to trauma, such as witnessing at an early age an ongoing pattern of violence between one's parents. The psychological impact of the traumatic experience depends both on the age at which it occurs and the duration of the trauma. In situations such as Margaret's, where the trauma continued over an extended period of time (decades in this case) and was experienced during the first decade of life, the damage is likely to be significantly greater (van der Kolk, 1996b).

We can see that Margaret displayed many of the features of this proposed condition: chronic affect dysregulation, difficulty controlling anger, self-destructive and suicidal behavior, dissociation, somatization, chronic guilt and shame, feelings of ineffectiveness, an inability to develop or maintain relationships with others, and a tendency to victimize others and to be revictimized herself. Her reliance on these mechanisms is not surprising in view of her history. Her inability to progress further in her development despite many years of therapy is also not surprising, because individuals in Margaret's situation often enlist their therapists' help in recreating their traumatic context, so that the therapist is seen as a rescuer, a victim, or a victimizer.

Therapy for such individuals experiencing these symptoms must help them see how their current stresses in life are experienced as a return to the traumas of their past (van der Kolk, 1989; Perry, Herman, van der Kolk, & Hoke, 1990), that is, how even while attempting to ride forward, they continue to look back and even to remain in the past. Cognitive behavioral therapy may be helpful in this regard. This technique focuses on helping the individual to identify "thinking errors," such as absolutist thinking, overgeneralization on the basis of isolated events, magnifying or minimizing the significance or extent of an occurrence, and focusing on only the negative elements in a situation ("selective abstraction") (Granvold, 1997). This approach also focuses on the client's identification of exaggerated expectations, and irrational beliefs. It is thought that this approach can help clients become more sensitive to their flawed thinking as it is happening, so that they can discount it and replace it with sounder conclusions (Granvold, 1997).

While Margaret's situation exemplifies an individual looking only towards the past while moving forward on a bicycle—that is, someone who has been unable to develop a future orientation—Douglas's experience illustrates what can happen when an individual lives in denial of the past while simultaneously attempting to develop a future orientation. Douglas is a gay African American man in his 40s. Although he was raised in the Deep South, he no longer lives there and only rarely visits his relatives there. His mother identifies as a Christian. She divorced his father because of his excessive drinking, his use of physical violence to gain his wishes, and his unexplained lengthy absences from their family home. Douglas's contact with his father following his parents' divorce was only slightly more infrequent than prior to the divorce. While growing up, he was apparently more effeminate than was acceptable to his siblings and his parents. His siblings attempted to "toughen" him up by embarrassing him in front of other family members and the church community. For instance, at one family event that occurred during Douglas's mid-adolescence, one of his brothers announced to the entire gathering that Douglas was the only one in the family who "had ever been fucked in the ass."

Rather than toughening him up and "making him a man," such experiences further deepened Douglas's sense of insecurity and distrust of others and exacerbated his already-existing difficulties with intimacy.

Unlike Margaret, Douglas is able on a certain level to plan for his future and to follow through with his plans. He has been consistently employed in responsible positions with insurance companies and research enterprises. Several years ago, he decided that he wanted to have a career, rather than only a sequence of various jobs. He received training as a medical assistant and now, while still working in that capacity, is pursuing more advanced training. He appears to be well-liked by the patients with whom he interacts.

On another level, though, Douglas has carried the wounds of his younger years with him, even as he refuses to acknowledge them and learn from those experiences. He continues to have difficulty with intimacy in relationships and even in choosing relationships wisely. He is not currently involved in a romantic relationship. All of his past sexual partners were discovered in clubs, where both the partners and Douglas were drinking heavily when they met. Each of these partners was a disappointment, and some of these encounters were disastrous. Several of the men were actually married and their wives did not know of their sexual activities with men; emotionally and physically, they were rarely available for a real relationship, and Douglas was but an easy mark for them. One, who had a propensity for violence, believed that tying Douglas to a bed and whipping him would be a good time for all. Each of these encounters further exacerbated Douglas's feelings of anger and distrust. Douglas built increasingly higher emotional walls around himself to protect himself, adopting the view that one should "Do unto others before they do unto you." Douglas perceived himself as the unfortunate victim of these encounters, all the while denying any responsibility for having created or entered into them.

There are few people in Douglas's life whom he calls friends. Those that he does have are periodically subjected to his outbursts of profanity and venom in response to perceived slights and offenses. It is as if he is testing them to see whether they are really friends or whether they, too, will hurt him as everyone else has. He has had intermittent difficulties with superiors at his various jobs as a result of his inappropriate challenges to their authority, resulting in reports to Human Resources for insubordination. Because Douglas never learned how to process his hurt and anger, he continues to display it in inappropriate ways. And, because he never processed and resolved the hurts and anger that he experienced while growing up, he is unable to evaluate each event or interaction as it is. Instead, every perceived injury is felt cumulatively with others that he has experienced in his lifetime, so that no event stands by itself as a single event in time. As a result, Douglas's actions and language are often disproportionate to the situation and, as such, are reactionary rather than responsive.

Douglas's use of alcohol allows him to momentarily forget the shame that he experiences each time he contemplates having sex with a man. Its use helps him to lower inhibitions and relieve feelings of guilt and anxiety related to internalized homophobia (Hicks, 2000; McKirnan & Peterson, 1989). Because he cannot allow himself to actively remember and process the shaming moments with his family, he is unable to move past those events and the feelings associated with them. Instead, he drowns the feelings out with alcohol and, because the alcohol also clouds his judgment, finds himself in situations that, at best, are awkward and at worst, potentially dangerous.

Even while Douglas is seemingly looking toward the future—a relationship, a job, a sexual encounter—he remains rooted in his past. He has compartmentalized his experiences and left them behind; he cannot learn from them and bring that knowledge forward with him on his bicycle to use in events of the present.

Douglas's way of dealing with life events and circumstances is reflective of an avoidant personality disorder (*DSM-IV-TR*, 2000). Douglas is unwilling to become involved with others unless he is sure that they will like him, and he is unable to have a truly intimate relationship because he is afraid of being shamed or ridiculed. He is hypersensitive to criticism, which has resulted in a severely restricted social network. Douglas remains unable to understand or identify personal boundaries, resulting in exposure to potentially dangerous situations with prospective intimates and in inappropriate confrontations with authority figures.

Cognitive or dialectical behavioral therapy may not be as helpful for Douglas as it might for Margaret. In contrast to Margaret, who thinks and talks only about events in her life that are long past, Douglas refuses to remember or discuss any situation actively. He is unable to identify situations that may trigger feelings of hurt or anger or fear because he has compartmentalized each experience. Narrative therapy has proven to be of limited value for the same reason; Douglas simply refuses to discuss any past event. It is only through the use of the bicycle metaphor that Douglas has been able to look back to identify strengths and abilities that he can use in the present and take with him into the future. He has not, as yet, however, been able to examine the situations from which he learned those strengths and abilities.

Unlike Geoffrey and Joseph, whose attention was focused, at least in part, on gaining control over their financial situations, Margaret and Douglas were concerned almost entirely with issues related to intimacy and the consequences of having witnessed or endured past emotional or physical abuse and trauma. Nevertheless, the bicycle metaphor may, over time, be a helpful prompt for individuals even in such circumstances. Consider Joshua's situation as an example. Joshua is an African American college student at a private university in the Midwest. Both of his parents are professionals with demanding careers. For several years, Joshua cut himself and purged after most meals. As Joshua was slowly reducing the frequency and intensity of his cutting and purging, we used the bicycle metaphor to look back to what he had experienced, what he had learned from those experiences, and what he could carry from it into his future. In one of our sessions, excerpted below, Joshua reflected on why he had cut and purged, what he had learned looking back at this episode in his life, and what knowledge he would carry forward with him as a result of his experience. He also spoke of what he would tell others who might learn from his experience.

> I would describe myself as lonely. I'm sick. Sickening. When I was growing up my sister looked this way, my brother looked this way. I was like one of a kind. I don't know any darker, dark kid previously so when I was growing up as a kid . . . it was funny because, like everybody, there's only like four dark people in my whole family so I was a darkie, yeah. I just think I'm sick.

> The only reason I cut myself is because I thought it would drain all the bad out of me, to make me feel a different type of way because, I don't know, it was stupid. I'll be sitting there and I was like, I can't take it, but let me try this and I just cut and while I was bleeding, I just feel some, I feel good. Like it's yes, that's how it's supposed to, it was like, I felt better when I was leaking. I didn't like being me. Okay, it was something, escape, it made me not be, or made me feel better about being, right?

> Even when I was younger I was gay . . . Then I used to puke because I didn't like the way I looked. That wasn't good either because, um, I always messed with boys, like I don't gain weight at all. Very skinny for my size. I can eat whatever I want to and still be skinny. I got hypoglycemia, like I always keep a snack on me or something. It was stupid. I don't see why I wanted to do it. Back then made me feel like I was feeling good. Like when it came out, it made all the pain inside come out with all the other stuff, so that's why I was into blood and cut myself. It was just I don't know, I don't know how to explain it.

> So reading them books, they was talking about people puking and cutting and I'm like, well, I can puke and I can cut. Maybe I feel like cutting me. They was looking fabulous in the magazines. Like, if you can puke and you can cut, you can look like that. Well, I feel like I can puke and cut. Well, see, that was killing me 'cause like I don't know it's stupid.

> I know I'm not stupid but doing that, that was somewhat stupid. 'Cause think about it, if I was just not paying no attention, pain and everything it

does, 'cause I was letting everything get, get to me. Like this was pissing me off and I couldn't say nothing because I was so young, so I would do this to myself or this happened during that day. I can't tell my parents because they weren't paying attention, so I feel the same way about just, it made me feel better about me when I was doing.

So what was bad inside? Being gay for god sakes. Back then I thought I was a three [on a scale of 10]. There wasn't nobody that ever told me I was ugly. I was always like, you're a cute kid and then I heard hot, sexy . . . I always heard it and I wasn't, for God sakes look at me, my lips are big, my nose is big, my head is very long, my body is very skinny.

So what made the change? Getting tired of it. Just was over it, hate it, like I can't just make me feel every day I want to do the same thing. You make me feel like forty-five minutes to an hour, all is said and done. I feel this way, that way, but then after a long while, you start looking at your arms and you start getting tracks and scrapes and people start asking. I just stopped doing, I just was fed up. I cut myself with a knife, it hurt, please give me a nice little nick okay.

So if there was a younger guy cutting or puking [I'd tell him], you don't need to, because at the end of the day, you're still going to feel that same way you did five minutes before you cut yourself. Ain't going to make you feel no type of difference. Going to give you more of a headache, make you miserable. You may think, you may seem like every time you do it you feel just a little bit better and you can't bear no more but you can. Think about it. Just think about it. In a situation like what, you said if you don't know what you're doing, if you cut, you can die or you bleed half out, now you go to the hospital and people looking at you like you trying to commit suicide. What you wanting to do? Puking early could tear up your esophagus. You'll learn, they'll learn. I've been doing that. The erosion of the throat, that, please, you don't know what that will do. The acid that comes up and goes back down. The erosion, I know you don't need to do it, it's not that serious, never was completely. At the end of the day, you're still going to be you and if people didn't like you, then they won't like you now, too, and that's what I think. If they make you feel that bad, stay away from them. That's what I do, I stay away from them . . . maybe you can stay whose company I can do without. That's a clue towards me.

People don't talk to kids, not like real talk to them. Like, basically, well, yeah, basically a kid wants somebody who can sit there and relate to what they do, been through, or going through. You can't sit there and try to sugar coat it.

Popping pills is like so ignorant. Trying to kill yourself with the pills . . . It's ignorant. 'Cause baby, that never worked. Okay, I'm not going to say it never worked, but it rarely works. You got to take a whole bottle of pills. Get that two and a half hour high. They're going to find you stroked in the middle of the bathroom in a puddle of spit. They're going to make you chew Vaseline, they're going to make you eat Vaseline. Lube you up with a, like four inch thick pipe, shove it down your throat and make you spit through her. Your throat is going to hurt for weeks on end because she has worked your esophagus. For what? Because you didn't like life that bad? Baby please! I never kill myself, I try to hurt myself, yes, that was stupid, but I ain't been to the extreme. Pop pills, or sniff something, or drink, I never did, oh, I started off, okay . . . I don't want to die, I want to hurt. Why do you want to hurt? Because I want to make myself feel. Basically I live to feel so that's why.

Joshua and I explored the path that he had taken on his metaphorical bicycle that had led him to cut and purge. Over time, I presented each of the following questions to Joshua for his consideration.

- What circumstances made you feel like cutting or purging? What made you feel like doing it less?
- Besides cutting and purging, what other ways did you use to deal with those circumstances?
- If you think back to what helped you deal with those situations besides cutting and purging, do you use any of these strategies now? When do you use them? How do you feel when you use them?
- If you look forward as you are riding your bicycle, what do you want to bring with you to help you if you should have these same feelings [sick, ugly] again? What would you like to leave behind?
- Can you imagine what those things you would like to leave behind might look like? Where would you like to leave them? How do you feel after you have left them there?
- Can you imagine what these things that you might want to bring with you might look like? How will you carry them? How do you feel while you are carrying them?

In encouraging Joshua to talk about his feelings in response to these questions, we focused both on his emotional feelings and how he felt in his body as he considered these possibilities. This focus on both the emotional and the physical feelings has helped Joshua to increase his awareness of the interconnectedness of his emotions and the sensations that he experiences in his body and develop new strategies to cope with feelings of anxiety, disgust, and shame.

Joshua has continued in college and has completely ceased cutting and purging. Although he had been self-hurting for several years, neither of his parents appeared to be aware of it. He utilized a transcript of one of our sessions together to initiate a dialogue with them about his cutting and his feelings about himself. Joshua has been able to identify both the feelings that trigger his urge to self-inflict wounds and alternative strategies to cope with these feelings. He has become a mentor of sorts to other young gay African American men who may be experiencing feelings of low self-worth and self-hate and speaks of his experience with them and his new-found strategies for managing his self-deprecatory feelings.

REFERENCES

American Psychiatric Association. (2000). *Diagnostic and statistical manual of mental disorders* (4th ed., text revision). Washington, DC: American Psychiatric Association.

Berger, D., & Berger, L. (1991). *We heard the angels of madness: A family guide to coping with manic depression.* New York: William Morrow.

Bremner, J. D., Randall, P., Scott, T. M., Bronen, R. A., Seibyl, J. P., Southwick, S. M., et al. (1995). MRI-based measures of hippocampal volume in patients with PTSD. *American Journal of Psychiatry, 152,* 973–981.

Elliott, T., Godshall, F., Shrout, J., & Witty, T. (1990). Problem solving appraisal, self-reported study habits, and performance of academically at-risk college students. *Journal of Counseling Psychology, 37,* 203–207.

Erikson, E. (Ed.). (1964). *Insight and responsibility.* New York: W. W. Norton & Company.

Erikson, E. (Ed.). (1968). *Youth and crisis.* New York: W. W. Norton & Company.

Erikson, E. H. (1997). *The life cycle completed.* New York: W. W. Norton & Company.

Gaa, J. (1979). The effect of individual goal setting conferences on academic achievement and modification of locus of control orientation. *Psychology in the Schools, 16,* 591–598.

Granvold, D. K. (1997). Cognitive-behavioral therapy with adults. In J. R. Brandell (Ed.), *Theory and practice in clinical social work* (pp. 164–201). New York: Free Press.

Hay, I., Byrne, M., & Butler, C. (2000). Evaluation of a conflict-resolution and problem-solving programme to enhance adolescents' self-concept. *British Journal of Guidance and Counselling, 28,* 101–113.

Heppner, P., Reeder, L., & Larson, L. (1983). Cognitive variables associated with personal problem-solving appraisal: Implications for counseling. *Journal of Counseling Psychology, 30,* 537–545.

Hicks, D. (2000) The importance of specialized treatment programs for lesbian and gay patients. In J. R. Guss & J. Drescher (Eds.), *Addictions in the gay and lesbian community* (pp. 81–94). New York: Haworth Medical Press.

Irwin, C. (1998). *Conquering the beast within: How I fought depression and won . . . and how you can, too.* New York: Random House.

McKirnan, D. J., & Peterson, P. L. (1989). Psychosocial and cultural issues in alcohol and drug abuse: An analysis of a homosexual community. *Addiction Behaviors, 14(5),* 555–563.

Miller, D., & Kelley, M. (1994). The use of goal setting and contingency contracting for improving children's homework performance. *Journal of Applied Behavioral Analysis, 27,* 73–84.

Nigro, G. (1996). Coping strategies and anxiety in Italian adolescents. *Psychological Reports, 79,* 835–839.

Perry, C. L., & Jessor, R. (1985). The concept of health promotion and the prevention of adolescent drug abuse. *Health Education Quarterly, 12,* 169–184.

Perry, J. C., Herman, J. L., van der Kolk, B. A., & Hoke, L. A. (1990). Psychotherapy and psychological trauma in borderline personality disorder. *Psychiatric Annals, 20,* 33–43.

Saxe, G. N., Vasile, R. G., Hill, T. C., Bloomingdale, K., & van der Kolk, B. A. (1992). SPECT imaging and multiple personality disorder. *Journal of Nervous and Mental Disease, 180,* 662–663.

Shakespeare, W. (2006). *As you like it.* (J. Dusinberre, ed.) London, UK: Thomson Learning.

Trammel, D., & Schloss, P. C. (1994). Using self-recording, evaluation, and graphing to increase completion of homework assignments. *Journal of Learning Disabilities, 7,* 75–82.

van der Kolk, B. A. (1989). The compulsion to repeat the trauma. *Psychiatric Clinics of North America, 12,* 389–411.

van der Kolk, B. A. (1996a). The body keeps score: Approaches to the psychobiology of posttraumatic stress disorder. In B. A. van der Kolk, A. C. McFarlane, & L. Weisaeth (Eds.). *Traumatic stress: The effects of overwhelming experience on mind, body, and society* (pp. 214–241). New York: Guilford Press.

van der Kolk, B. A. (1996b). The complexity of adaptation to trauma: Self-regulation, stimulus discrimination, and characterological development. In B. A. van der Kolk, A. C. McFarlane, & L. Weisaeth (Eds.). *Traumatic stress: The effects of overwhelming experience on mind, body, and society* (pp. 182–213). New York: Guilford Press.

SUGGESTIONS FOR FURTHER READING

Alcohol and Alcoholism

Barr, A. (1999). *Drink: A social history of America.* New York: Carroll & Graf Publishers Inc.

Heather, N., & Robertson, I. (2000). *Problem drinking* (3rd ed.). New York: Oxford University Press.

Cutting/Purging

Gordon, R. A. (2000). *Eating disorders: Anatomy of a social epidemic* (2nd ed.). Malden, MA: Blackwell Publishers Ltd.

Walsh, B. W. & Rosen, P. M. (1988). *Self-mutilation: Theory, research, treatment.* New York: Guilford Press.

Family Violence

Holden, G. W., Geffner, R., & Jouriles, E. N. (Eds.). (1998). *Children exposed to marital violence: Theory, research, and applied issues.* Washington, DC: American Psychological Association.

Thorne-Finch, R. (1992). *Ending the silence: The origins and treatment of male violence against women.* Toronto, Canada: University of Toronto Press.

CHAPTER 3

The Doughnut:

Finding Focus

THE IMPORTANCE OF FOCUS

Focus, or attention, can be thought of as the mechanisms that we utilize to prepare to process stimuli, turn our attention to what is to be processed, and determine how far to process it (Heilman, Watson, Valenstein, & Goldberg, 1987). Attention is critical because it determines what enters into our information-processing system and because individuals are believed to be able to pay attention to only a finite amount of information at any given time (Ashcraft, 1989). Without attention or focus, we lose the ability to filter out what is not of importance and attend to the information that we may truly need.

As children, we learn about the importance of paying attention or focusing from any number of sources. For instance, Aesop's fable of the hare and the tortoise teaches us the value of focus and perseverance. In that fable, the hare challenges the tortoise to a race to the finish line. The hare becomes distracted from his goal and is eventually passed by the tortoise. Ultimately, the hare loses the race to the tortoise, who moved much more slowly than the hare but remained focused on the task at hand (Aesop, 1947).

OBSTACLES TO FOCUS

Any number of situations may cause an individual to be inattentive or impulsive, resulting in a lack of focus. Symptoms of various mental illnesses, such as major depression, certain anxiety disorders, and bipolar disorder may include impulsivity and inattentiveness. Feelings of anxiety (as distinct from symptomatology of an anxiety disorder), symptoms of attention-deficit/hyperactivity disorder

(ADHD), dementia, brain injury, or the effects of an ingested substance such as crack cocaine or methamphetamine, may also induce impulsivity and lack of attention. Individuals may also be unable to focus because they feel overwhelmed by their circumstances and the multiple demands that they face in their lives.

This chapter focuses on the use of a metaphor to address impulsivity and a lack of focus that is remediable in whole or in part through the use of verbal therapies and behavioral techniques. Because it is beyond the scope of this chapter to review all such conditions, a more detailed discussion is limited to depression, generalized anxiety disorder, bipolar disorder, and ADHD as examples of conditions in which a lack of attention or focus may be addressed in part through the incorporation of metaphor.

Depression

Sadness is a part of the human condition. Everyone experiences sadness or feels depressed at some time for some reason—a disappointment, a loss, a frustration. That is not the same, though, as the experience of major depression. As one client diagnosed with major depression explained to me, "You can say when you are sad that you feel blue. But when you have depression, you feel nothing. You don't know blue. You don't see color anymore."

The client was not far from the truth. There is, indeed a biochemical basis for major depression. The classical model of major depression attributes the illness to an imbalance of the neurotransmitters norepinephrine and serotonin in the brain (Schwartz & Schwartz, 1993). It is thought that the occurrence of major depression depends on the interaction of this biochemical imbalance with an individual's pre-existing vulnerability, stress, and existing personal resources (Mrazek & Haggerty, 1994). More recent research suggests greater complexity in the development of depression (Duman, Malberg, Nakagawa, & D'Sa, 2000; Fujita, Charney, & Innis, 2000).

What distinguishes depression from sadness, from a feeling of being depressed? A *major depressive episode* is characterized by a period of at least two weeks during which the individual experiences a depressed mood or a lack of pleasure or interest in nearly all things (*Diagnostic and Statistical Manual of Mental Disorders,* 4th ed., text revision; *DSM-IV-TR*; American Psychiatric Association, 2000). Symptoms may include having no feelings, feeling anxious, or feeling sad; increased irritability; social withdrawal; severely reduced or increased appetite; being unable to sleep (insomnia) or sleeping too much (hypersomnia); psychomotor changes such as an inability to sit still or slowed speech, thinking, and body movements; decreased energy and increased fatigue; and a sense of worthlessness or guilt. Individuals may think of committing suicide or may attempt to do so.

Unlike a feeling of being depressed, a diagnosis of major depression requires that the individual be experiencing a clinically significant degree of impairment in social, occupational, or other important areas of functioning. Not infrequently, this impairment in functioning is attributable to a great extent to the individual's impaired abilities to think, concentrate, make decisions, and remember, which are additional symptoms of major depression.

Numerous strategies exist for the treatment of depression; they may be used singly or in combination. These include antidepressant medications and various forms of verbal therapy, such as psychotherapy, behavioral therapy, cognitive-behavioral therapy, and brief insight therapy (Beck, 1967; Schwartz & Schwartz, 1993). The use of electroconvulsive therapy, once widely relied upon for the treatment of depression (cf. Beck, 1967), has become controversial because of its overuse and misuse and the complications associated with its use (Fink, 1999). The use of metaphor can be integrated into most forms of verbal therapy.

Anxiety and Anxiety Disorders

Like depression, anxiety is a part of the human condition. William Shakespeare, in *The Merchant of Venice,* aptly described anxiety as "Your mind is tossing on the ocean" (Act I, scene I, line 8). Anxiety may be a healthy response to an existing threat or danger, preparing the body to fight or flee, or it may be due to a conflict, such as between one's internal values and externally imposed demands or between one's own contradictory values. Unlike depression, however, which derives from a focus on events of the past, anxiety results from a focus on future-anticipated events, which may or may not occur. In some circumstances, individuals may also experience depression at the prospect of being unable to control the future in order to avoid the feared occurrence.

Under some circumstances, anxiety may actually be helpful to the individual. For example, a low level of anxiety about a test may motivate a student to prepare better to do well. However, higher levels of anxiety may interfere with an individual's ability to process information from his or her environment accurately (Clark & Beck, 1989; Coles, Turk, Heimberg, & Fresco, 2001) and may lead to symptoms such as rapid breathing (Gilbert, 2002), a feeling of tightness in the chest (Frankel, 2001), a loss of appetite, sweating (Heurtin-Roberts, Snowden, & Miller, 1997; Hoehn-Saric & McLeod, 1993; May, 1977; McLeod & Hoehn-Saric, 1993), and an inability to focus attention (Fox, 1993; Mathews, May, Mogg, & Eysenck, 1990). Individuals who experience high levels of anxiety may focus on thoughts that are not relevant to the task at hand (Ingram & Kendall, 1987) and may perceive a situation as threatening even when no threat actually exists (Eysenck, 1991; Mathews & MacLeod, 1994; Wells & Papageorgiou, 1998).

The feeling of anxiety results from the interaction of various systems including the brain stem nuclei, the limbic system, the prefrontal cortex, and the cerebellum. The brain stem is partly responsible for controlling arousal, while the limbic system is that part of the brain that controls our emotional and autonomic responses to stressors. The prefrontal cortex is responsible for cognitive assessment, planning, and decision making and, as such, can modify responses to stimuli that provoke fear (Fuster, 1989; Pohl & Gershon, 1990).

Although the experience of anxiety may be near-universal, the development of an anxiety disorder is not. Some scholars believe that anxiety disorders that are directed to a specific object, such as a fear of certain places, result from a conditioned avoidance response (Hall & Lindzey, 1957; Mowrer, 1951).

Generalized anxiety disorder, which is the focus of this discussion, is to be distinguished from specific phobias and from panic attacks and panic disorder. Generalized anxiety disorder (GAD) is characterized by the occurrence of excessive worry for a preponderance of days during a six-month period and difficulty controlling the worry, which is not directed to a specific occurrence or physical complaint, as in a specific phobia or panic attack, and is not due to the physiological effects of a substance or other medical condition (*DSM-IV-TR*, 2000). The adult suffering from GAD must experience at least three of six symptoms, resulting in clinically significant distress or impaired functioning in social, occupational, or other arenas of life: restlessness, easy fatigability, difficulty in concentrating, irritability, muscle tension, and sleep disturbance.

Margaret, whom you may remember from Chapter 2, had been diagnosed with bipolar disorder, but she also suffered from generalized anxiety disorder. Because she was always worried about what the future would hold and what trauma or catastrophe might occur, she was unable to find any peace or to enjoy even small moments of pleasure. Because she was constantly worried about almost everything, she was unable to focus on a specific task or to make a decision about a particular matter.

Treatment for generalized anxiety disorder may consist of one or more approaches: medication, psychoeducation about the nature of the anxiety disorder, and some form of psychological intervention (Andrews et al., 1994; Roemer & Orsillo, 2005). The optimal form(s) of treatment for any particular individual depends on the type of anxiety disorder that the individual has and the severity of his or her symptoms. Metaphors can be used in conjunction with many forms of psychological intervention.

Bipolar Disorder

A diagnosis of bipolar disorder requires that the individual have experienced one or more manic or hypomanic episodes, with or without having experienced a depressive episode (*DSM-IV-TR*, 2000). The individual may or may not also experience a major depressive episode to be diagnosed with bipolar disorder.

A manic episode consists of a period of at least one week in duration, or less if hospitalization is necessary, during which the individual's mood is persistently elevated, expansive, or irritable. An individual with an elevated or expansive mood must experience three or more of the following symptoms to be diagnosed with mania, while an individual experiencing an abnormally irritable mood must experience four: an inflated self-esteem or grandiosity; a decreased need for sleep; distractibility, evidenced by an inability to filter out irrelevant stimuli; flight of ideas or the sense that his or her thoughts are racing; speech that is pressured, rapid, loud, and often hostile or angry; increased involvement in goal-directed activities or psychomotor agitation, evidenced by pacing and restlessness; and excessive involvement in activities that may be pleasurable but that have a high potential for painful or negative consequences, such as buying sprees, reckless driving, and indiscriminate sexual behavior.

A hypomanic episode is also characterized by these features, but, in contrast to a manic episode, hallucinations or delusions cannot be present. Additionally, the abnormal mood need persist only four days for a diagnosis of hypomania, in contrast to the week-long duration required for a diagnosis of mania (*DSM-IV-TR*, 2000). In order for an individual to be diagnosed with either mania or hypomania, his or her symptoms cannot be attributable to the effects of a substance or general medical condition and must result in significant impairment or distress in an important area of functioning, such as employment or family life.

Individuals with untreated mania may progress through several distinct stages (Bowden, Kusumakar, MacMaster, & Yatham, 2002). Stage I, which is comparable to hypomania, is characterized by a euphoric mood, irritability if demands are not satisfied, overconfidence and grandiosity, coherent but often tangential thoughts, a preoccupation with religion or sex, racing thoughts, an increased rate of speech and psychomotor activity, and an increase in spending, telephone usage, and smoking.

When I met Sabrina, a client in a therapy group for individuals with bipolar disorder, she was exhibiting behavior indicative of hypomania. Sabrina was a single white woman in her early 20s who was employed as a technician at a major medical institution. She consistently interrupted others in group, insisting that her experiences and insights were more valuable and instructive than those of the other group members or any of the various therapists. She exaggerated the importance of her contributions to her workplace supervisors and spent much of her time outside of work and therapy engaged in shopping sprees, resulting in ever-increasing credit card balances that her income could not support.

Katy's behavior is illustrative of the symptoms of the second stage of mania. During the second stage of mania, individuals may become openly hostile and aggressive and/or depressed, may experience delusions, have increased psychomotor acceleration and pressure of speech, and may engage in assaultive behavior. Katy was a middle-aged white woman who described herself as very religious, intelligent, and hard-working. She had refused any and all treatment for her bipolar disorder, believing that "there was nothing wrong" except for others' unrelenting persecution of her. Her illness gradually worsened, resulting in severe disruption to her work and to her relationships and interactions with others. She believed that government agents were following her in an attempt to acquire enough evidence against her to discredit her. Unfamiliar persons were perceived as threats. Ultimately, Katy attacked a woman who had attempted to be of assistance to her, in the belief that she was protecting herself from possible assault by a government interrogator.

During the third and most severe stage of mania, individuals are often hopeless, panic-stricken, and incoherent. They frequently are not oriented to time and place and may experience bizarre delusions, hallucinations, or both and engage in frenzied psychomotor activity (Bowden et al., 2002). The actress Patty Duke, who suffered from bipolar disorder, said of her manic phases, "When the mania starts to ebb and you return to the planet, you begin to recognize that you have done some very strange things" (Duke & Hochman, 1992, p. 17).

There is a genetic component involved in the development of bipolar disorder. Individuals tend to develop the disorder during early adulthood and, because of the nature of the illness, are often at elevated risk for difficulties in employment, family life, and school. There is also an increased risk of suicide attempts and completed suicide (Miles, 1997). Bipolar disorder is treatable, but not curable, with appropriate medication (Yatham, Kusumakar, & Kutcher, 2002) and psychosocial interventions (Bauer, 2002), which may utilize metaphors.

Attention-Deficit/Hyperactivity Disorder (ADHD)

ADHD is characterized by "a persistent pattern of inattention and/or hyperactivity-impulsivity that is more frequently displayed and more severe than is typically observed in individuals at a comparable level of development" (*DSM-IV-TR*, 2000, p. 85). Although some symptoms of the disorder must have been present prior to the age of seven years, some individuals may not be diagnosed with this disorder until they are much older. Also, to be diagnosed with ADHD, the individual must experience the symptoms for at least six months and display impairment in at least two domains of functioning, such as home life and employment.

Individuals with ADHD may appear to be inattentive or careless with school work or in their occupational functions. They are often unable to complete one task before initiating another one, and they often experience difficulty in organizing tasks and activities. Because of these difficulties, they may try to avoid tasks that require sustained attention and effort. Individuals with ADHD may often become distracted by irrelevant stimuli and interrupt their ongoing tasks to attend to external noises and events that others are able to disregard. Inattention may be evidenced through forgetfulness, frequent shifts in the topic of conversation, and a failure to attend to details. Hyperactivity in adolescents and adults is often expressed as restlessness and an inability to engage in relatively quiet activities.

THE METAPHOR

The metaphor of the doughnut is a simple one: "Keep your eye on the doughnut, not the hole." Despite the seeming simplicity of this metaphor, it can be utilized with clients on several levels.

At the most basic level, a doughnut is round, has a hole in the center, and, more often than not, is sweet to the taste. To receive any benefit from the doughnut, one must focus on the doughnut; focusing on the hole will fail to satisfy any hunger pangs. Also, because most doughnuts are sweet, the individual consuming the doughnut most likely will derive at least a short-term feeling of pleasure. Focus on a particular task or object, then, may ultimately lead to pleasure.

On a more profound level, use of the doughnut metaphor allows the individual to step back and focus his or her attention as a witness or observer to the process. This stepping back will, in turn, help the individual to reduce the level of his or her reactivity and, ultimately, reduce the likelihood that the individual will perpetuate his or her unrewarding and potentially self-destructive or unproductive behavior.

Because the doughnut has a circular form, and the circle is universally known and has many associations, numerous variations of the doughnut metaphor are possible. These can be introduced by the counselor or therapist or by the client. For example, consider the following objects, all of which have circular form: the halo, a symbol of holiness; the ring, a symbol of unity and faithfulness; the entwined double circles of the symbol of infinity; the wheel, a symbol of mobility; the wheel of dharma, a common symbol of Buddhism, whose motion signifies the continuous spread of Buddha's teachings and whose eight spokes represent the eightfold path of Buddha; the circle dance of Shiva Nataraja, the Lord of the Dance, the Hindu god of destruction and rebirth; the compass, providing direction; the eye, representing the spiritual gateway to the soul; the symbol for yin and yang, signifying the masculine and feminine aspects; and the mandala, which is evident in various forms, each with its distinct concept and purpose, such as healing (Cornell, 2006; Tucci, 2001).

I use the doughnut metaphor in my work with individuals who have a difficult time focusing as a symptom of depression, generalized anxiety, or lesser levels of mania. After presenting the metaphor, I ask individuals to explain what they think this means and how it might relate to their particular situation. This analogy has proven to be helpful to a number of individuals, as illustrated below.

USING THE METAPHOR

Tamara, an African American woman in her 20s, was only recently diagnosed with bipolar disorder. When she was 15, her mother ejected her from the household at the behest of her stepfather, who found her difficult and uncooperative. She was hospitalized for three months following a suicide attempt. Upon discharge, she participated in an intensive outpatient program for emotionally disturbed and troubled youth but was discharged from the program once she reached the age of 18. Since that time, she has been involved in several short-lived same-sex relationships, some of which have been as abusive as her relationship with her mother and stepfather. More recently, she has been involved with a woman several years her senior, who has helped her to obtain steady employment and who encourages her to participate in counseling and adhere to a medication regimen to equilibrate her mood swings.

Tamara has been on probation for over a year as the result of damage to property caused by a woman who borrowed her car. At the time, Tamara did not carry auto insurance and was unable to pay for the cost of repairs. Her probation officer informed her that the police had been unable to find the woman responsible and, as a result, Tamara would be required to pay the four-figure sum in order to be released from probation. Alternatively, she would be sentenced to time in jail.

Tamara was overwhelmed by what she perceived as the enormity of the problem and was initially unable to formulate any possible solution. She had only recently begun to work full-time and was concerned with moving to a new apartment and having a commitment ceremony with her partner.

I used the metaphor of the doughnut with Tamara and her partner, Chantelle. What was the doughnut here, and what was the hole? They both agreed that the doughnut was finding a solution to the problem of the restitution, successfully completing probation, and moving on with life to more pleasant events and possibilities. Chantelle quickly worked out a budget utilizing both of their incomes and discovered that together they would be able to pay the entire restitution in approximately two months. That would mean pushing back their plans for a new apartment and for their commitment ceremony. Chantelle was able to convince Tamara that the delay was irrelevant in the bigger picture; in other words, focusing on the delay was really focusing on the hole, instead of on the doughnut.

I also used the doughnut metaphor with Joseph. (For additional details about Joseph's situation, see Chapter 5.) Joseph had suffered several major depressive episodes in the past and was currently dysthymic at the time he consulted me. Joseph had been raised by his maternal grandmother and continued to live with her as a young adult. As he described her, she was controlling, negative, and relatively uneducated.

Joseph's room was located in the attic of his grandmother's house. One day, he returned home from his work to find that she had removed his bed from his room and had moved it to another room in the house, which she planned to rent out in order to have some additional cash. She entered Joseph's room with a rake, threatening to rake up and throw out anything that was on the floor, which included his books for his college courses. Joseph was scheduled to take an exam in one of his courses that morning, but, afraid that his grandmother would destroy his property, he cleaned his room instead of going to his college course. He arrived at his class too late to take his exam and was required to take a make-up test.

Joseph's hurt and anger were apparent when he related this episode to me. However, he had difficulty delineating any possible courses of action that he could take in the future that might prevent a recurrence of this scenario. Direct questions to Joseph about possible ways to handle his situation brought forth only angry and/or presently unrealistic solutions: "Get rid of the bitch!" "Find another place and leave!" This prompted me to use, instead, the metaphor of the doughnut to help Joseph identify what he considered important and what demanded his primary attention. I posed this question to him: "Are you up to trying an experiment here? Sometimes experiments work and sometimes they don't. Let's see what happens with this one." After receiving

Joseph's somewhat reluctant approval to proceed, I asked, "Suppose we look at the situation here like a doughnut. If you try to eat the hole, you end up with nothing, so you have to focus on the doughnut to get anything of substance. What here is of substance for you? What is your doughnut, the thing that you really want?"

Joseph decided that the "doughnut" was his time and succeeding in his college courses, which would be necessary if he were to graduate with a degree and establish a more stable living situation for himself. The "hole" was engaging in a power struggle with his grandmother and responding to her in a manner designed to ensure an escalation of their confrontation. He concluded that his grandmother was unlikely to modify her behavior with him, especially since it had been consistent over many decades with both him and with her adult children. However, he could modify his approach to the situation. Joseph brainstormed strategies to minimize the likelihood that the situation would recur: installing a lock on his bedroom door; safeguarding those possessions that he considered valuable, rather than leaving them in piles on the floor; and, ultimately, saving sufficient funds to be able to afford his own apartment.

Veronica, an African-American woman in her mid-30s, had been diagnosed with bipolar disorder. Her past aggressive behavior had resulted in several arrests and short-term stays in the city jail. At the time of our work together, she was participating in group therapy for individuals recently discharged from hospital treatment for bipolar disorder and major depression.

During one group session, Veronica expressed her frustration with her gynecologist. She had recently gone for a pelvic examination and Pap test, her first in many years. The doctor had discovered a lump in her breast while performing the accompanying breast examination. Consistent with established guidelines for mammograms for women in Veronica's age group, he had referred her for mammography. The results of that examination confirmed the existence of a lump, but its specific nature remained unclear. The physician had then referred her for a biopsy, which she had undergone approximately 10 days prior to this group session. Veronica had telephoned her physician's office several times in an attempt to obtain the results of that biopsy, but had been unable to reach the doctor and her calls had not been returned.

As Veronica spoke, she became increasingly agitated and angry. She bellowed her intention to present herself to her physician's assistant at the medical office and demand her test results, promising to "punch her lights out" if her demands were not immediately gratified. Knowing Veronica's past history, the possibility that she would approach the situation in this manner was all too real.

I introduced the metaphor of the doughnut and then asked Veronica what the doughnut might represent in her particular situation. She identified the conversation with the doctor as her ultimate goal. Members of the group quickly jumped in, pointing out that it was not merely a dialogue with the doctor that was needed, but a conversation in which he presented the biopsy results to her and explained their meaning and significance and potential courses of action. Veronica agreed with this observation.

We proceeded to role play Veronica's intended visit to her doctor's office, with Veronica playing herself and another woman in the group assuming the role of the office receptionist. Although Veronica was somewhat calmer than her earlier diatribe had suggested she might be, her approach to the "receptionist" was still accusatory, confrontational, and vituperative. A male member of the group jumped in to replace Veronica and assume her role.

This second "Veronica" began to assuage the "receptionist's" feelings, sympathizing with her about the difficulties and stresses inherent in her job responsibilities and complimenting her on her professional manner with patients, despite their sometimes unreasonable behavior. Veronica interjected angrily that she was "not about to kiss anyone's ass." The group reminded her that the receptionist very likely had little control over the doctor's schedule or the release of the test results and Veronica's goal (the doughnut) was to learn and understand the implications of the biopsy results, not to win an argument with the receptionist or to obtain from her an acknowledgment of what Veronica felt was the physician's inattentiveness and lack of concern for her situation. In essence, the group pointed out, Veronica would have a greater likelihood of success in accomplishing her goal if she were able to enlist the receptionist as an ally, rather than alienating her as an enemy.

Veronica resumed the role play as herself and practiced integrating this recommended approach to the receptionist. Several days later, Veronica came to the group all smiles and beaming. She had successfully negotiated with the receptionist to arrange a meeting with her gynecologist. The success of her attempt had surprised Veronica. In her mind, her efforts were doubly rewarded with the news that the biopsy had been negative and the lump that had been detected was a large cyst.

REFERENCES

Aesop. (1947). *Aesop's fables*. New York: Grosset & Dunlap.

American Psychiatric Association. (2000). *Diagnostic and statistical manual of mental disorders* (4th ed., text revision). Washington, DC: American Psychiatric Association.

Andrews, G., Creamer, M., Crino, R., Hunt, C., Lampe, L., & Page, A. (1994). *The treatment of anxiety disorders: Clinician's guide and patient manuals*. Cambridge, UK: Cambridge University Press.

Ashcraft, M. (1989). *Human memory and cognition.* Glenview, IL: Scott, Foresman.

Bauer, M. S. (2002). Psychosocial interventions for bipolar disorder: A review. In M. Maj, H. S. Akiskal, J. J. Lopez-Ibor, & N. Sartorius (Eds.), *Bipolar disorder* (pp. 281–313). New York: John Wiley & Sons, Ltd.

Beck, A. T. (1967). *Depression: causes and treatment.* Philadelphia: University of Pennsylvania Press.

Bowden, C. L., Kusumakar, V., MacMaster, F. P., & Yatham, L. N. (2002). Diagnosis and treatment of hypomania and mania. In L. N. Yatham, V. Kusumakar, & S. P. Kutcher (Eds.), *Bipolar disorder: A clinician's guide to biological treatments* (pp. 1–16). New York: Brunner-Routledge.

Clark, C. R., & Beck, A. T. (1989). Cognitive theory and therapy of anxiety and depression. In P. C. Kendall & D. Watson (Eds.), *Anxiety and depression: Distinctive and overlapping features* (pp. 379–411). San Diego, CA: Academic Press.

Coles, M. E., Turk, C. L., Heimberg, R. G., & Fresco, D. M. (2001). Effects of varying levels of anxiety within social situations: Relationship to memory perspective and attributions in social phobia. *Behaviour Research and Therapy, 39,* 651–665.

Cornell, J. (2006). *Mandala: Luminous symbols for healing.* Wheaton, IL: The Theosophical Publishing House & Quest Books.

Duke, P., & Hochman, G. (1992). *A brilliant madness: Living with manic-depressive illness.* New York: Bantam Books.

Duman, R. S., Malberg, J., Nakagawa, S., & D'Sa, C. (2000). Neuronal plasticity and survival in mood disorders. *Biological Psychiatry, 48,* 732–739.

Eysenck, M. W. (1991). Cognitive factors in clinical anxiety: Potential relevance to therapy. In M. Briley & S. E. File (Eds.), *New concepts in anxiety* (pp. 418–433). Boca Raton, FL: Macmillan.

Fink, M. (1999). *Electroshock: Restoring the mind.* New York: Oxford University Press.

Fox, E. (1993). Attentional bias in anxiety: Selective or not? *Behaviour Research and Therapy, 31,* 487–493.

Frankel, B. L. (2001). "Chest pain" in patients with anxiety disorders. In J. W. Hurst & D. C. Morris (Eds.), *Chest pain* (pp. 415–428). Armonk, NY: Futura Publishing Company.

Fujita, M., Charney, D. S., & Innis, R. B. (2000). Imaging serotonergic neurotransmission in depression: Hippocampal pathophysiology may mirror global brain alterations. *Biological Psychiatry, 48,* 801–812.

Fuster, J. M. (1989). *The prefrontal cortex.* New York: Raven Press.

Gilbert, C. (2002). Interaction of psychological and emotional effects with breathing dysfunction. In L. Chaitow, D. Bradley, & C. Gilbert (Eds.), *Multidisciplinary approaches to breathing pattern disorders* (pp. 111–129). London: Harcourt Publishers Limited.

Hall, C. S., & Lindzey, G. (1957). *Theories of personality.* New York: John Wiley.

Heilman, K. M., Watson, R. T., Valenstein, E., & Goldberg, M. E. (1987). Attention: Behavioral and neural mechanisms. In V. B. Mountcastle (Ed.), *Handbook of physiology: Section 1. The nervous system* (pp. 461–481). Bethesda, MD: American Physiological Society.

Heurtin-Roberts, S., Snowden, L., & Miller, L. (1997). Expressions of anxiety in African-Americans: Ethnography and the Epidemiological Catchment Area Studies. *Culture, Medicine, and Psychiatry, 21,* 337–363.

Hoehn-Saric, R., & McLeod, D. R. (1993). Somatic manifestations of normal and pathological anxiety. In R. Hoehn-Saric & D. R. McLeod (eds.), *Biology of anxiety disorders* (pp. 177–222). Arlington, VA: American Psychiatric Publishing, Inc.

Ingram, R. E., & Kendall, P. C. (1987). The cognitive side of anxiety. *Cognitive Therapy Research, 11,* 523–536.

Mathews, A., & MacLeod, C. (1994). Cognitive approaches to emotion and emotional disorders. *Annual Review of Psychology, 45,* 25–50.

Mathews, A. M., May, J., Mogg, K., & Eysenck, M. (1990). Attentional bias in anxiety: Selective search or defective filtering. *Journal of Abnormal Psychology, 99,* 166–173.

May, R. (1977). *The meaning of anxiety* (rev. ed.). New York: W. W. Norton & Company, Inc.

McLeod, D. R., & Hoehn-Saric, R. (1993). Perception of physiological changes in normal and pathological anxiety. In R. Hoehn-Saric & D. R. McLeod (Eds.), *Biology of anxiety disorders* (pp. 223–244). Arlington, VA: American Psychiatric Publishing, Inc.

Miles, C. P. (1997). Conditions predisposing to suicide: A review. *Journal of Nervous & Mental Diseases, 164,* 231–246.

Mowrer, O. H. (1951). Two-factor learning theory: Summary and content. *Psychology Review, 58,* 350–354.

Mrazek, P. J., & Haggerty, R. J. (Eds.). (1994). *Reducing risks for mental disorders: Frontiers for preventive intervention research.* Washington, DC: National Academy Press.

Pohl, R., & Gershon, S. (Eds.) (1990). The biological basis of psychiatric treatment. In *Progress in basic clinical pharmacology* (pp. 1–33). Basel, Switzerland: Karger.

Roemer, L., & Orsillo, S. M. (2005). An acceptance-based behavior therapy for generalized anxiety disorder. In S. M. Orsillo & L. Roemer (Eds.), *Acceptance and mindfulness-based approaches to anxiety: Conceptualization and treatment* (pp. 213–240). New York: Springer.

Schwartz, A., & Schwartz, R. M. (1993). *Depression: Theories and treatments: Psychological, biological and social perspectives.* New York: Columbia University Press.

Shakespeare, W. (1992). *The merchant of Venice* (B. A. Mowat & P. Werstine, Eds.). New York: Washington Square Press.

Tucci, G. (2001). *The theory and practice of the mandala.* Mineola, NY: Dover Publications.

Wells, A., & Papageorgiou, C. (1998). Social phobia: Effects of external attention on anxiety, negative beliefs, and perspective taking. *Behavior Therapy, 29,* 357–370.

Yatham, L. N., Kusumakar, V., & Kutcher, S. P. (2002). *Bipolar disorder: A clinician's guide to biological treatments* (pp. 1–16). New York: Brunner-Routledge.

SUGGESTIONS FOR FURTHER READING

Anxiety

Capps, L., & Ochs, E. (1995). *Constructing panic: The discourse of agoraphobia.* Cambridge, MA: Harvard University Press.

Dozier, R. W., Jr. (1998). *Fear itself.* New York: St. Martin's Press.

Self-efficacy

Bandura, A. (1997). *Self-efficacy: The exercise of control.* New York: W. H. Freeman and Company.

Maddux, J. E. (Ed.). (1995). *Self-efficacy, adaptation, and adjustment: Theory, research, and application.* New York: Plenum.

CHAPTER 4

The Snowflake:

Achieving Self-Actualization

SELF-ACTUALIZATION

The importance of self-actualization has been recognized throughout time. Judaism teaches:

> In life, you discover that people are called by three names: One is the name the person is called by his father and mother; one is the name people call him, and one is the name he acquires for himself. The best one is the one he acquires for himself (Siegel, 1983).

William Shakespeare wrote in *Hamlet*, "To thine own self be true" (Act I, scene iii, line 78). What, then, does it mean to acquire one's own name and to be true to oneself?

Being true to oneself and acquiring one's own name, that is, one's own identity, can be thought of as being self-actualized. Abraham Maslow (1970, p. 150) defined self-actualization as "the full use and exploitation of talents, capacities, potentialities." According to Maslow, self-actualized individuals are characterized by qualities such as creativity, spontaneity, autonomy, a sense of humor, a capacity for deep interpersonal relationships, humility and respect for others, strong ethical standards, a sense of appreciation and wonder, a need for privacy, self-acceptance, and an accurate perception of reality. Maslow (1959, 1970) also indicated that self-actualized persons are more likely to focus on universal and social rather than personal problems, identify and sympathize with humanity, and have mystical experiences.

In addition, Maslow found that self-actualized persons often reported having had life-changing experiences, which he called peak experiences, during which the ego boundary loosened and the individual felt a sense of union with other beings, with nature, and with the divine (Maslow, 1970).

Individuals were often challenged to integrate these brief but intense experiences into their lives. In contrast, nadir experiences, which could also prompt individuals to examine their sense of identity and their world view, often occur in conjunction with a crisis, such as a medical emergency or a death. A third form of transpersonal experience, which Maslow termed the plateau experience, is characterized by a sense of happiness and contentment. Self-actualized individuals, Maslow found, are able to integrate these peak, nadir, and plateau experiences into their daily lives.

Maslow (1970) hypothesized that individuals are not able to become self-actualized unless they are first able to satisfy more basic needs. The very bottom rung of this hierarchy of needs consists of biological and physiological needs, such as hunger and thirst, followed by safety needs. Attachment, the next rung, refers to our need to be loved and to love. Attachment is followed successively in this hierarchy by fulfillment of cognitive needs, such as knowledge, understanding, and novelty; aesthetic needs, such as order and beauty; and, towards the top of the hierarchy, self-actualization. Maslow placed the need for transcendence, or religious and spiritual needs, at the very pinnacle of the hierarchy. Although some scholars have criticized Maslow's specific ordering of needs in the hierarchy (Neher, 1991), the existence of these domains of need and the concept of self-actualization are widely acknowledged (Hagerty, 1999; Ventegodt, Merrick, & Andersen, 2003).

The development of self-actualization implies the recognition and further development of each individual's talents and attributes and their creative use. This means that an individual's present state of growth can be judged against his or her potential for growth. It should not be taken to mean that individuals should be compared against other individuals or that an individual who is perceived as more complex than another is necessarily more likely to be self-actualized.

Just as each individual is unique with respect to a particular combination of personality traits, talents, attributes, and life experiences, so too is each snowflake unique in its shape and/or journey earthward so that no two snowflakes are the same (Roach, 2007). For this reason, I have found that the metaphor of the snowflake is useful in discussing the concept of self-actualization with clients.

THE METAPHOR OF THE SNOWFLAKE

An examination of the similarities between snowflakes and people may be helpful to understand why the snowflake might work as a metaphor in counseling. Snow is actually a form of atmospheric ice that is formed following the evaporation of water off of a supercooled droplet in a cloud and the condensation of the vapor onto an ice crystal in the same cloud without first passing through a liquid phase (Gosnell, 2005). Snow crystals can take any of more than 80 basic forms, including columns, needles, stellars, plates, and irregular shapes. In fact, there are 10,000,000,000,000,000,000 molecules in a typical snow crystal, so that the number of ways in which they could be arranged is unimaginable (Gosnell, 2005). Similarly, although individuals may bear a superficial resemblance to each other in terms of their physical appearance and personalities, they may actually be quite different. This is true even of identical twins, who look alike but whose personalities, preferences, and attitudes may be quite different.

In their journey to earth, snow crystals may have fallen as far as six miles and may have encountered a variety of conditions. Mariana Gosnell (2005, p. 423) described the perils inherent in a snow crystal's descent through the atmosphere to earth:

> Water droplets may stick to it and form bumps of rime. Winds may break off one branch [of the snow crystal], or three, or five. Other crystals may hit it and become attached. It may descend in a spiral path, with one edge angled more into the airstream than the others, and since a leading edge grows faster than a trailing edge (having more water vapor available to it), a crystal that holds this orientation could end up developing only one arm.

Each such change in the snowflake's environment will cause a change in its growth and development (Libbrecht, 2006). Not surprisingly, the snow crystal that arrives on earth may look markedly different from the way it did when it was first created. Much as with humans, the history of the snowflake's growth determines what its ultimate shape will be.

Temperature is a critical determinant of the snowflake's shape (Libbrecht, 2005). When the weather is slightly below freezing, the snow crystals will be plate-like. If it becomes slightly colder, slender columns and needles will be formed (Libbrecht, 2006). High humidity will produce snow crystals that are complex and branched, while lower levels of humidity result in snow crystals that are simpler and faceted.

"Temperature" is similarly critical to the development of individuals. A lack of human warmth and responsiveness towards a child may cause the child significant distress, particularly if the absence of affection and attention is prolonged (Polansky, 1982; Seiner & Gelfand, 1995; Solantaus-Simula, Punamaki, & Beardslee, 2002; Spitz, 1945, 1946). When the environment is too "hot," on the other hand—that is, when it is characterized by excessive anger or violence—the child may grow up to be a victim or a victimizer, to injure himself or herself or others, or to be unable to recognize and respect the boundaries that exist in healthy relationships (Fagan & Browne, 1994).

Snowflakes often display many facets, which are flat crystalline surfaces. The growth of facets is an important factor in the development of the different shapes and patterns among snowflakes. Reflections off of these facets give snow its sparkle. Similarly, each individual possesses different dimensions of his or her personality. People may display different aspects of themselves in different situations so that in some contexts they may "sparkle," while in other environments they may appear lackluster.

The development of facets is a stabilizing process, resulting in flat surfaces and simple shapes. The formation of branches, known as branching, occurs when a small bump appears on the surface of the crystal. Because the bump protrudes further in the supersaturated air than the area surrounding it, water molecules will accumulate faster at the site of the bump. These bumps will develop into branches, and additional branches will then form off of them. In contrast to facets, branching creates more complexity in the snowflake structure but also brings with it increased instability (Libbrecht, 2003).

If we compare the snowflake's process of development to human development, we see that, like more developed snowflakes, self-actualized persons within Maslow's framework have had both their basic biological and physiological needs and their attachment needs fulfilled. Their complexity and self-actualization derives from their ability to integrate their "branching" peak and nadir experiences into their lives.

Sometimes, snowflakes develop what is called "knife-edge instability," whereby the snow crystal forms a sharp edge. This increases the crystal's growth, which, in turn, sharpens the edge even more. This can be likened to what Maslow termed a nadir experience, which can prompt the individual to examine his or her world view and self-identity.

USING THE METAPHOR

Just as we can focus on the unique characteristics of a single snowflake or on the process by which it developed, so too can clients utilize the metaphor of the snowflake in any number of ways. Some clients may use the metaphor to reflect their feelings, while others may find it helpful to identify the qualities that they believe make them who they are or to contemplate the factors that have influenced their development and the trajectory of their growth.

I have introduced the metaphor of the snowflake by suggesting that visualizing oneself as a snowflake or the journey that one might make as a snowflake might be a relaxing way to begin a session. I then describe briefly how snowflakes are formed and their journey to earth, much as I have done above, but in a more abbreviated fashion. I then invite the client or clients to close their eyes and imagine what they would be like as a snowflake, or what their journey to earth might be like, or what might happen once they arrive on the earth as a snowflake. (I have found that clients are often more open to visualizing themselves as snowflakes, and that it is easier to do so, if winter is actually approaching or if there is already snow on the ground.) The following examples illustrate how several clients participating in a group session for adults with bipolar disorder and major depression utilized the snowflake metaphor.

Heather, a woman in her 40s, had been a dynamic and well-respected professional in her field prior to the onset of her depression. Her symptoms of depression—an overwhelming feeling of sadness, lack of energy, feelings of worthlessness, an inability to concentrate—gradually worsened to the point that she was no longer able to work or even to care for herself. Following a period of hospitalization, she participated in both group and individual therapy sessions and followed a medication regimen designed to alleviate her symptoms. Although she had once been able to manage a household in addition to her high-pressure job, Heather was unable to do so even after her hospitalization, and she moved in with some of her adult siblings. After a prolonged period during which her symptoms failed to diminish, it became clear that she would never be able to return to her previous employment because of the passage of time and the resulting atrophy of her professional skills.

Heather used the snowflake metaphor as a way to express her feelings about her then-current situation, stating "There is only blackness, blackness all around me. I feel nothing. I am just part of the crowd, nothing. I am just a clump." When asked to describe what she might see as a snowflake falling to earth, Heather repeated, "Blackness. Nothing. Just blackness all around me." Heather could not see herself as a snowflake; she could only see darkness and blackness around her as she fell. As Heather continued to describe her journey and arrival on earth as a snowflake, it became apparent that she could not see any color. She had no sense of boundary and embodiment as a snowflake, but was "just there," in her words. Heather's description revealed the depth of her depression and her inability to see outside of it. The use of the snowflake metaphor enabled her to express in words what she had not been able to verbalize previously. Her newly found ability to put these feelings into words both surprised and relieved her. Now, she could label with words what she had been feeling.

Emily was startled by the idea of the snowflake metaphor, exclaiming, "This is deep!" Emily was in her early 20s at the time and had had to take a leave of absence from her job in order to attend group therapy sessions as part of the treatment plan for her bipolar disorder. Her image of herself as a snow-flake was quite different than Heather's. Emily saw herself as the embodiment and reflection of multiple colors, saying "I reflect light, joy. It is like my heart, light." Emily suggested that individuals immediately prior to their deaths must be like a snowflake, reflecting light and color before they ultimately fade and die. Emily's description of Emily-as-snowflake as multiply colored light that was reflected "all over" mirrored her seemingly pressured and rapid speech and elevated level of impatience that was suggestive of hypomania.

Candace was also in her 20s and had been participating in this ongoing group for several weeks. She described Candace-as-snowflake as having many branches and sharp edges, and indicated that she was like her snowflake be-cause she, too, had many edges that she used to keep people away and to protect herself. Her snowflake shape was symmetrical but jagged, and she mounted an offense as she fell towards the earth from the clouds, pushing other snowflakes away. I asked her how the snowflake's fall was similar to her own life journey. Candace responded, "The best defense is a good offense."

Candace's answer and her description of herself as a snowflake were con-sistent with her family members' accounts of Candace's interactions with them and with individuals who had once been her friends but had distanced them-selves from her because of what they believed were unwarranted emotional attacks against them. Despite Candace's seeming acknowledgment of her role in these interactions with this depiction of a snowflake, Candace continued to deny that anything that she had said or done could have prompted individu-als to withdraw from their involvement with her. Rather, she asserted, they did so because she was unique and different in a strange and magnificent way. She then suggested that her snowflake was different from all of the others and that she liked being different, that she didn't care if other people looked at her and thought that she was strange.

Each of the individuals focused on a different aspect of themselves as a snowflake: Heather on what she saw outside of herself, that is, her fall; Emily, the color, and Candace, the shape. Each such depiction of themselves as a snowflake or their description of their journey as a snowflake would require significantly more discussion than could take place in the context of a 50-minute group session that had been attended by eight individuals. However, the snowflake metaphor allowed them to express sentiments that they had until then been unable to share and provided insight into the issues that could be addressed in future individual sessions.

I have also used the snowflake metaphor in sessions with individual clients. Geoffrey, whose situation is described in greater detail in Chapter 5 as well as other chapters, was diagnosed with schizophrenia when he was in his late 30s, although it is likely that he had been experiencing the symptoms of the illness for some time prior to his formal diagnosis by a psychiatrist. Geoffrey used the metaphor of the snowflake to describe both his then-current view of himself and how he wanted others to see him. His mother, he informed me, had always said that he was an old soul. He decided that if he were a snowflake, he would be part of a glacier that had been in existence for thousands of years. He described Geoffrey-as-snowflake as complex, with multiple dimensions, facets, and branches, reflecting the complexity of Geof-frey-as-person. We used this description as the basis to begin discussing the many complexities of Geoffrey's personality and existence as he saw them. Geoffrey continued with an explanation of how he as Geoffrey-the-snowflake related to others around him:

> I am part of the glacier that represents gays and lesbians. We are not part of the water that constitutes the larger society. We are frozen, dismissed, seen as not worthy and different. When we are fully accepted by society, the glacier will dissolve and we will be part of the water, part of the larger society and seen the same way as everyone else.

Geoffrey's description of himself as a component of a glacier served as a starting point from which to explore his feelings of marginalization by his family and society in general, his need to develop an enlarged support system, and his desire to be more connected to the larger gay community in his city of residence.

Joseph, described in Chapter 5 and various other chapters, was an African American man in his 20s who self-identified as gay. Joseph had been diag-nosed with dysthymia, although it appeared that he had suffered at least one major depressive episode years earlier. Joseph said of Joseph-the-snowflake:

> I wonder what shape I would be. I would enjoy the cool breeze against me as I fell to earth. I would have many sides, because I am moody. I would be big, bigger than the other snowflakes, and observe everything. I would land someplace different, where I never know anything. I would be social with the other snowflakes. It would be scary because I don't know the other snowflakes. You have to hold your own.

I asked Joseph whether he ever felt like that now. He proceeded to tell me about the recent death of a friend of his who, he said, "was one of the few [Joseph] ever met who completely understood him, no judgment. He was always there, genuinely interested." Joseph then talked about how the idea of himself as a snowflake had made him think of his friend's death at the age of 33, and how, like the snowflake, his friend had died after such a short lifetime. The idea of the snowflake prompted Joseph to think about his own life and the possibility that he might die young without ever having attained his goals.

Joseph then spoke of the importance of controlling his depression, which, he said, could keep him from achieving his dreams and lead to an early death, metaphorically:

> It feels so good not to be depressed. I have stuff to do, I'm not focused on what I don't have. Depression keeps you from moving forward, depression keeps you from doing anything that gets you out of the depression. You have to not allow depression to control you and rationalize so that you recognize every fault you have and feel that there's nothing you can do about it. Then you sabotage yourself and let it eat away at you.

We talked about what it meant to Joseph to "hold his own." He felt that he could never show any sign of vulnerability; he had to be "bigger." To be respected, to "hold his own," he had to develop a persona and a "rep" that said: "If you mess with me, I'll kill you." This stance helped Joseph remain alive amidst the violence in his family and his neighborhood, but, paradoxically, it also increased his fear that someone would "take him out" in order to establish their own "rep" and command "respect." It also interfered with his efforts to secure and retain employment and to interact in social strata outside of the one in which he lived.

Joseph then compared himself to a snowflake and, as with him, how difficult it is for an individual snowflake to be recognized apart from all of the other snowflakes. He continued,

> All my life I wanted to be in my 20s and now it's almost over. I want to be able to admire what I've done with my life. The thought of it eats away at me, the possibility of not getting recognition. I made a decision to be an openly gay [musician]. I don't want to live the typical [musician's] lifestyle with girls and cars, messed up, that. There are no gay [musicians] with respect and credibility.

The use of the snowflake metaphor can be used in conjunction with art therapy. (Art therapy is discussed in greater detail in Chapter 12.) Materials such as paper, scissors, glitter, and paste can be made available at the beginning of an individual or group session. After describing the nature of snowflakes, the client(s) can be invited to use the materials that have been provided to make a snowflake that reflects who they are and/or their journey to earth. Clients can then be invited to share their descriptions of themselves-as-snowflakes or their journeys as snowflakes to the counselor/therapist and with other group members, if it is being done in a group session. The focus on the resulting art product and its description may create for some individuals a needed distance that will reduce the threat they experience in exploring themselves and/or their situations.

Masaru Emoto (2006) has suggested that the image of water crystals together with selected musical excerpts can be useful in alleviating stress and reducing bodily pain. His work in this regard offers the possibility of introducing another variation of the snowflake metaphor, particularly with individuals who are unfamiliar with snow but can see or feel water. The metaphor of the water or snow crystal can be introduced to an individual client or group together with a musical selection. The clients can be asked to use the music and the image together to visualize who/what they are or who/what they would like to be as a water or snow crystal moving in response to the musical vibration. Alternatively, the clients can be invited to select an excerpt of music that reflects their image of themselves as a water or snow crystal or that embodies their journey from the sky to the earth.

The augmentation of the metaphor experience with musical excerpts may enhance individuals' understanding of their own emotional responses. Music stimuli has been shown to facilitate the experience and identification of emotion (Thaut, 1990); create a condition that promotes the client's disclosure of his or her problems, feelings, and thoughts (Harper & Bruce-Sanford, 1989); facilitate an understanding of others' emotional communications; and help individuals to synthesize, control, and modulate their own emotional behavior (Thaut, 1990). Because of these properties, music has been used effectively in both therapeutic and educational settings to promote individual growth, insight, and learning and to effectuate behavioral change (Bunt, 1988). There is also literature to suggest that music may serve a therapeutic function among individuals with severe mental illness, including overall reduction in psychotic symptoms, reduction in negative symptoms of schizophrenia, improved social functioning and increase in subjective sense of community participation, decreased social isolation and increased level of interest in external events (Gold, Heldal, Dahle, & Wigram, 2005; Hayashi et al., 2002; Talwar et al., 2006; Tang, Yao, & Zheng, 1994).

REFERENCES

Bunt, L. (1988). Music therapy: An introduction. *Psychology of Music, 16,* 3–9.

Emoto, M. (2006). *Water crystal healing: Music & images to restore your well-being.* New York: Atria Books.

Fagan, J., & Browne, A. (1994). Violence between spouses and intimates: Physical aggression between women and men in intimate relationships. In A. J. Reiss, Jr., & J. A. Roth (Eds.), *Understanding and preventing violence: Volume 3, Social influences.* Washington, DC: National Academy Press.

Gold, C., Heldal, T. O., Dahle, T., & Wigram, T. (2005). Music therapy for schizophrenia or schizophrenia-like illnesses. *Cochrane Database Systems Review, 2,* CD004025.

Gosnell, M. (2005). *Ice: The nature, the history, and the uses of an astonishing substance.* Chicago: University of Chicago Press.

Hagerty, M. R. (1999). Testing Maslow's hierarchy of needs: National quality-of-life across time. *Social Indicators Research, 46(3),* 249–271.

Harper, F. D., & Bruce-Sanford, G. C. (1989). *Counseling techniques: An outline and overview.* Alexandria, VA: Douglass Publishers.

Hayashi, N., Tanabe, Y., Nakagawa, S., Noguchi, M., Iwata, C., Koubuchi, Y. et al. (2002). Effects of group musical therapy on inpatients with chronic psychoses: A controlled study. *Psychiatry and Clinical Neurosciences, 56,* 187–193.

Libbrecht, K. (2003). *The snowflake: Winter's secret beauty.* St. Paul, Minnesota: Voyageur Press.

Libbrecht, K. G. (2005). The physics of snow crystals. *Reports on Progress in Physics, 68,* 855–895.

Libbrecht, K. (2006). *Ken Libbrecht's field guide to snowflakes.* St. Paul, Minnesota: Voyageur Press.

Maslow, A. H. (1959). Creativity in self-actualizing people. In H. H. Anderson (Ed.), *Creativity and its cultivation* (pp. 83–95). New York: Harper & Row.

Maslow, A. H. (1970). *Motivation and personality* (2nd ed.). New York: Harper & Row.

Neher, A. (1991). Maslow's theory of motivation: A critique. *Journal of Humanistic Psychology, 31,* 89–112.

Polansky, N. A. (1982). *Integrated ego psychology.* New York: Aldine.

Roach, J. (2007). "No two snowflakes the same" likely true, research reveals. *National Geographic News.* Retrieved October 15, 2007, from http://nationalgeographic.com/news/2007/02/070213-snowflake_2.html

Seiner, S. H., & Gelfand, D. M. (1995). Effects of mothers' simulated withdrawal and depressed affect on mother-toddler interactions. *Child Development, 66,* 1519–1528.

Shakespeare, W. (1992). *Hamlet.* (C. Hoy, Ed.) New York: W. W. Norton & Company.

Siegel, D. (1983). *Where heaven and earth touch: An anthology of Midrash and Halacha.* Spring Valley, NY: Town House Press.

Solantaus-Simula, T., Punamaki, R.-L., & Beardslee, W. (2002). Children's responses to low parental mood. II: Associations with family perceptions of parenting styles and child distress. *Journal of the American Academy of Child & Adolescent Psychiatry, 41(3),* 1519–1528.

Spitz, R. (1945). Hospitalism: An inquiry into the genesis of psychiatric conditions in early childhood. *The Psychoanalytic Study of the Child, 1,* 53–74.

Spitz, R. (1946). Hospitalism: A follow-up report. *The Psychoanalytic Study of the Child, 2,* 113–117.

Talwar, N., Crawford, M. J., Maratos, A., Nur, U., McDermott, O., & Procter, S. (2006). Music therapy for in-patients with schizophrenia: Exploratory randomized controlled trial. *British Journal of Psychiatry, 189,* 405–409.

Tang, W., Yao, X., & Zheng, Z. (1994). Rehabilitative effect of music therapy for residual schizophrenia: A one-month randomized controlled trial in Shanghai. *British Journal of Psychiatry, Suppl. 24*, 38–44.

Thaut, M. H. (1990). Neuropsychological processes in music perception and their relevance in music therapy. In R. F. Unkefer (Ed.), *Music therapy in the treatment of adults with mental disorders* (pp. 3–32). New York: Schirmer Books.

Ventegodt, S., Merrick, J., & Andersen, N. J. (2003). Quality of life theory III. Maslow revisited. *The Scientific World Journal, 3*, 1050–1057.

SUGGESTIONS FOR FURTHER READING

Art Therapy Exercises

Buchalter, S. I. (2004). *A practical art therapy.* London: Jessica Kingsley Publishers.

Malchiodi, C. A. (2002). *The soul's palette: Drawing on art's transformative powers.* Boston: Shambala Publications, Inc.

Simmons, L. L. (2006). *Interactive art therapy: "No talent required" projects.* Binghamton, NY: Haworth Press, Inc.

Mindfulness and Visualization

Gawain, S. (2002). *Meditations: Creative visualization and meditation exercises to enrich your life.* Novato, CA: Nataraj Publishing.

Kabat-Zinn, J. (1994). *Wherever you go there you are: Mindfulness meditation in everyday life.* New York: Hyperion.

CHAPTER 5

The Elephant And The Blind Men:

Learning New Perspectives

ROLES AND ROLE TRANSFORMATION

As individuals grow, they are assigned and acquire multiple roles, that is, social categories or positions, each of which is imbued with a set of expected behavior patterns. Some of these roles may be ascribed on the basis of various characteristics or traits, such as age or socioeconomic status. Others may be acquired by choice or as the result of individual accomplishment. The writer Antoine de Saint-Exupéry observed, "One is a member of a country, a profession, a civilization, a religion. One is not just a man" (Wartime Writings 1939–1944, quoted in de Saint-Exupéry, 2002, p. 43).

Each of these various and diverse roles, memberships, and identities may bring widely varied obligations and rights. For instance, the obligations of an adult child to his or her family in his or her capacity as a child are significantly different from those of the same adult in his or her role as "parent" and "breadwinner" for his or her own children. Similarly, one's role as a member of a profession, such as law, medicine, or counseling, confers vastly different rights and responsibilities than does one's role as a next-door neighbor.

A number of scholars have maintained that the assumption of multiple roles is, in general, beneficial to individuals. A more complex self-structure, that is, defining oneself in relation to a larger number of domains or a large number of attributes, may help to protect individuals from emotional turmoil (Linville, 1982, 1987). Individuals with multiple roles are believed to benefit psychologically and materially, as well as in their interpersonal dealings with others (Barnett, 1999; Barnett, Marshall, & Singer, 1992; Repetti, Matthews, & Waldron, 1989; Waldron, Weiss, & Hughes, 1998).

However, the assumption of multiple roles may lead to role strain caused by difficulties meeting the obligations and demands inherent in each role. As an example, many women in their 40s and 50s may experience role strain as the result of conflicting demands on their necessarily limited time and energy that are occasioned by the diversity and intensity of their various roles: wife or partner, mother of small children, daughter of aging and ill parents, employee, supervisor of others, churchgoer, and so forth. These multiple roles may engender not only strain but also conflict, if contradictory expectations exist between roles or if there are inconsistencies inherent in any of the individual roles. It is believed that much of the role strain that women face is attributable to the failure of workplaces and families to adapt to changing economic and social realities (Scharlach, 2001; Silverstein, 1991; cf. O'Neil & Greenberger, 1994).

Yet another perspective focuses on the context in which an individual fulfills one or more roles, rather than attending to only the number of roles that the individual inhabits (Moen, Dempster-McClain, & Williams, 1989; Voydanoff & Donnelly, 1999). For instance, individuals who receive role support for a particular role from individuals who are significant to them are more likely to find the role rewarding than an individual in essentially the same role who receives no support from others (Stephens & Townsend, 1997).

Various circumstances may affect individuals' ability to continue successfully in roles that they have assumed, to transform the nature of the roles that they have assumed, or to transition to new roles. Retirement, for instance, may bring an end to one's role as an employee or employer but usher in a new role as a tutor for inner-city children struggling to learn to read. It is likely that all individuals will experience role loss at multiple points of their lives, simply as a function of aging and the demands and responsibilities that are successively acquired and lost and acquired as one moves from childhood into adolescence and into adulthood (Meyer, 2007).

Some role losses, however, result from circumstances that are neither predictable nor controllable, such as mental illness. Individuals who experience acute episodes of severe mental illness may lose multiple roles simultaneously: life partner, parent, employee, employer, friend, driver. Individuals who once considered themselves and were thought of by others as independent may find themselves in a dependent role. Frequently, such role losses are accompanied by shock, anger, and grief.

In such circumstances, I have used the story of the blind men and the elephant as a vehicle to discuss with the client the implications of the role loss and how the client can integrate the loss into his or her life situation in a positive manner. This exploration can focus on the client's continuing ability to address one or more dimensions of the various demands inherent in a given role; the client's redefinition of a "lost" role or of himself or herself in order to continue in that role; and/or the discovery and establishment of new roles to replace those that have been lost as a result of the mental illness.

THE STORY OF THE BLIND MEN AND THE ELEPHANT

You may remember the story of the blind men describing the elephant. Each man was standing at a different part of the elephant, and each believed that what he "saw" with his hands was the complete whole. That story actually comes from the following poem that was written by John Godfrey Saxe.

It was six men of Indostan
To learning much inclined,

Who went to see the Elephant
(Though all of them were blind),

That each by observation
Might satisfy his mind.

The First approached the Elephant,
And happening to fall

Against his broad and sturdy side,
At once began to bawl:

"God bless me! but the Elephant
Is very like a wall!"

The Second, feeling of the tusk,
Cried, "Ho! what have we here,

So very round and smooth and sharp?
To me 'tis mighty clear

This wonder of an Elephant
Is very like a spear!"

The Third approached the animal,
And happening to take

The squirming trunk within his hands,
Thus boldly up and spake:

"I see," quoth he, "the Elephant
Is very like a snake!"

The Fourth reached out an eager hand,
And felt about the knee.

"What most this wondrous beast is like
Is mighty plain," quoth he;

"'Tis clear enough the Elephant
Is very like a tree!"

The Fifth, who chanced to touch the ear,
Said: "E'en the blindest man

Can tell what this resembles most;
Deny the fact who can,

This marvel of an Elephant
Is very like a fan!"

The Sixth no sooner had begun
About the beast to grope,

Than, seizing on the swinging tail
That fell within his scope,

"I see," quoth he, "the Elephant
Is very like a rope!"

And so these men of Indostan
Disputed loud and long,

Each in his own opinion
Exceeding stiff and strong,

Though each was partly in the right,
And all were in the wrong!

There is a final verse, less often heard, that informs us of the moral of the story:

So oft in theologic wars,
The disputants, I ween,

Rail on in utter ignorance
Of what each other mean,

And prate about an Elephant
Not one of them has seen!

Just as the blind men "saw" different aspects of the elephant, believing that what they saw constituted the entire elephant, so too do we see that the elephant has been endowed with various meanings in diverse cultures and faiths. The elephant has been used in Buddhism to signify the strength of the mind, as well as the aspiration, effort, intention, and analytic ability of the Buddha. Elephants were sometimes used to adorn stupas, monuments constructed as symbols of faith; the elephants symbolized the strength of the mind of a Buddha.

Hindu art reveals yet other meanings of the elephant. Elephants were variously used as symbols of rain clouds and as the keepers of darkness, the symbols of ignorance (Elgood, 1999). However, the elephant also bore even greater significance in the context of the Hindu religion. According to legend, the god Siva (also known as Shiva), the lord of destruction and renewal, came to see his wife Parvati. The figure of a young boy blocked his entrance to her doorway. Not realizing that the figure was that of his own son, Siva beheaded him. Parvati was stricken with grief and rage and threatened to destroy the heavens and the earth. Siva promised to bring the head of the first living being that he saw, which was the elephant. The head of the elephant was placed on the lifeless body of the young boy, who came alive. The son of Parvati was given the name Ganesha, from *gana* (followers of Siva) and *isha* (lord). Lord Ganesha is commonly depicted with the head of an elephant and with four or more hands, each holding a symbol. The elephant head symbolizes auspiciousness, strength, and intellectual prowess. Lord Ganesha is revered as the guardian of doorways and the remover of obstacles, "the Lord of the Beginnings" (Elgood, 1999).

The blindness of the men who seek to understand the nature of the elephant has also been imbued with symbolic value that can be utilized as a metaphor. There are numerous references in the New Testament to blindness that provide a foundation. For instance, Matthew 14:14 alludes to the Pharisees as blind men and notes the folly of the blind leading the blind, stating "If a blind man leads a blind man, both will fall into a pit." In Matthew 20:29–34, we see that blindness is essentially equated with the need for redemption by Christ:

> As Jesus and his disciples were leaving Jericho, a large crowd followed him. Two blind men were sitting by the roadside, and when they heard that Jesus was going by, they shouted "Lord, Son of David, have mercy on us!"
>
> The crowd rebuked them and told them to be quiet, but they shouted all the louder, "Lord, Son of David, have mercy on us!"
>
> Jesus stopped and called them. "What do you want me to do for you?" he asked.
>
> "Lord," they answered, "we want our sight."
>
> Jesus had compassion on them and touched their eyes. Immediately they received their sight and followed him.

Not surprisingly in view of this passage, blindfolding has been used as a symbol of spiritual blindness, darkness born of ignorance (Hall, 1979).

USING THE METAPHOR

I have introduced this metaphor to clients both individually and when working with a group by suggesting that a relaxing and yet productive way of beginning a session might be to read a poem and then to discuss its relevance for the clients who are present. I have then read the poem and asked clients how they thought it might be relevant to their lives in general or to their current situations. I have found that clients have used this metaphor in any number of ways.

Geoffrey, for instance, compared the many aspects of the elephant to the number of roles that he had assumed or been given during his life. As an example, some of the roles that he mentioned included brother, son, boyfriend, trophy wife (to his former long-term same-sex partner), instructor, and friend. We used these observations to begin to explore how the various roles overlapped and how they were distinct from each other, consistencies and inconsistencies between the roles and his self-portrayal in each of these roles, and the extent to which Geoffrey could or would be willing to integrate these various aspects of himself into a cohesive whole. Geoffrey felt strongly that complete consistency and integration across all of the diverse roles would never be possible, since the majority of his family members were neither supportive nor accepting of his homosexuality and, in their efforts to "convert" him to heterosexuality, admonished him that he "could do anything he set his mind to," intimating that he could become heterosexual and have sex with women if he just "set his mind" to it. The use of the metaphor, however, helped Geoffrey to reflect on the extent to which greater cohesiveness could be achieved and strategies that he could use to accomplish this.

Joseph, on the other hand, appeared to relate more strongly to the idea of blindness. When I first presented the poem to him, he was immediately struck by how he had been "blind" to the way he had been living his life and to his true character and behavior. Joseph indicated that he had always thought of himself as reliable, trustworthy, and tough. Additionally, he thought of the world as an evil place in which someone was always trying to best him. Indeed, Joseph's view of life was that it was a continuous battle, with no reprieve.

Joseph stated that the metaphor prompted him to think about what might be in front of him that he was unable to see because of his metaphorical blindness. He was startled to see his own pattern of unreliability and even more shocked when he discovered that he had been "blind" to acts of kindness that had been shown to him by various individuals in his network of friends and acquaintances, who seemingly had no underlying motive other than to assist him.

Leon, a young African American man whom I saw in a group for men, used the metaphor in a way that was completely different. The group had been discussing romantic relationships and the criteria that each individual used to determine whether a partner or prospective partner truly loved and respected them. Leon began to describe how he had suffered abuse at the hands of a previous partner. The varying views of the elephant became, first, the numerous ways in which he had rationalized that his partner really loved him despite the abuse and, subsequently, the many strategies that an individual could use in order to extricate him- or herself from an abusive relationship.

Delilah, a single woman in her twenties, was a participant in a group for individuals with bipolar disorder and major depression. Delilah had previously discussed the high level of anxiety she suffered each evening when she returned to her apartment and was there by herself. The silence and solitude, she said, would cause her "to freak out" and lead to all-night episodes of eating and pacing.

Delilah and other group members used the elephant metaphor to identify various mechanisms that could be used to reduce Delilah's level of anxiety. They were quite concrete with their analogy; each part of the elephant was used to depict a particular strategy. As an example, the elephant's trunk became the vacuum cleaner hose; Delilah could use her time productively to clean the apartment, which, by her own description, was "a disaster." The elephant's ears became Delilah's ears, and she could use her ears to listen to relaxing music that would help her to calm down and drift off to sleep.

As seen, clients have used the metaphor of the elephant and the blind men to identify strategies for handling various situations (role conflict, termination of relationships, sleeplessness, and anxiety) and the nature of their "blindness." Clients could also potentially use the metaphor to identify strategies that they could use to overcome their "blindness" and maintain or regain their "sight." The metaphor could be used in conjunction with role playing by an individual or members of a group. Each "role" or "blind man" could represent a different perspective of a given situation; the elucidation of varying perspectives may help clients reframe their own understanding of the event or situation in question.

REFERENCES

Barnett, R. C. (1999). A new work-life model for the twenty first century. *The Annals of the American Academy of Political and Social Science, 562,* 143–158.

Barnett, R. C., Marshall, N. L., & Singer, J. D. (1992). Job experiences over time, multiple roles, and women's mental health: A longitudinal study. *Journal of Personality and Social Psychology, 62,* 634–644.

de Saint-Exupéry, A. (2002). *A guide for grown-ups: Essential wisdom from the collected works of Antoine de Saint-Exupéry.* San Diego, CA: Harcourt, Inc.

Elgood, H. (1999). *Hinduism and the religious arts.* London: Cassell.

Hall, J. (1979). *Dictionary of subjects and symbols in art.* Boulder, CO: Westview Press.

Linville, P. W. (1982). Affective consequences of complexity regarding the self and other. In M. S. Clark & S. T. Fiske (Eds.), *Affect and cognition* (pp. 79–110). Hillsdale, NJ: Erlbaum.

Linville, P. W. (1987). Self-complexity as a cognitive buffer against stress-related illness and depression. *Journal of Personality and Social Psychology, 52,* 663–676.

Meyer, W. (2007). Role loss. In S. Loue & M. Sajatovic (Eds.). *Encyclopedia of Aging and Public Health* (pp. 729–730). New York: Springer.

Moen, P., Dempster-McClain, D., & Williams, R. M. (1989). Social integration and longevity: An event history analysis of women's roles and resilience. *American Sociological Review, 54,* 635–647.

O'Neil, R., & Greenberger, E. (1994). Patterns of commitment to work and parenting: Implications for role strain. *Journal of Marriage and the Family, 56,* 101–118.

Repetti, R. L., Matthews, K. A., & Waldron, I. (1989). Employment and women's health: Effects of paid employment on women's mental and physical health. *American Psychologist, 44,* 1394–1401.

Scharlach, A. E. (2001). Role strain among working parents: Implications for workplace and community. *Community, Work, & Family, 4,* 215–230.

Silverstein, L. B. (1991). Transforming the debates about child care and maternal employment. *American Psychologist, 46,* 1025–1032.

Stephens, M. A. P., & Townsend, A. L. (1997). Stress of parent care: Positive and negative effects of women's other roles. *Psychology and Aging, 12*(2), 376–386.

Voydanoff, P., & Donnelly, B. W. (1999). Multiple roles and psychological distress: The intersection of worker, spouse, and parent roles with the role of the adult child. *Journal of Marriage and the Family, 61,* 725–738.

Waldron, I., Weiss, C. C., & Hughes, M. E. (1998). Interacting effects of multiple roles on women's health. *Journal of Health and Social Behavior, 39,* 216–236.

SUGGESTIONS FOR FURTHER READING

Gender and Role

Disch, E. (Ed.). (2003). *Reconstructing gender: A multicultural anthology* (3rd ed.). Boston, MA: McGraw-Hill.

Kimmel, M. S. (2000). *The gendered society.* New York: Oxford University Press.

Metaphorical Blindness

Freud, A. (1966). *The ego and mechanisms of defense.* New York: International Universities Press.

Thich Nhat Hanh. (2001). *Anger: Wisdom for cooling the flames.* New York: Riverhead Books.

Strategies for Problem Solving

Covey, S. R. (1989). *The 7 habits of highly effective people*. New York: Simon & Schuster.

McGraw, P. C. (1999). *Life strategies: Doing what works, doing what matters*. New York: Hyperion.

CHAPTER 6

The Ladder:

Measuring Growth

STAGES OF DEVELOPMENT AND GROWTH

In Chapter 2, we briefly discussed in conjunction with the bicycle metaphor the model for human development that was formulated by Erik Erikson. In that chapter, we focused specifically on the development of a future orientation during the period of adolescence. In this chapter, we consider Erikson's complete model of psychosocial development and how that model can be used in conjunction with the metaphor of the ladder both to assess the client's current stage of development and to measure change during the course of longer-term therapy or counseling.

Erikson hypothesized that psychosocial growth and development occurs in stages, each of which is associated with a psychosocial crisis (Erikson, 1997). In this context, a "crisis" is conceived of as "a turning point for better or worse" (Erikson, 1964, p. 139), to which the individual can respond either adaptively or maladaptively. The extent to which an individual is able to resolve each such crisis successfully depends upon his or her experiences during earlier stages of development. Accordingly, each stage marks the development of a different facet of the individual's identity in relation to the external social world; the component parts of the individual ultimately give rise to the whole individual (known as epigenetic theory). The successful resolution of the crisis at a particular stage of development results in the development of a basic psychological strength or virtue at that stage. Let us now consider each hypothesized stage.

Stage 1: Infancy. During infancy, the extent to which the child's caregivers, such as parents, meet the child's physical and psychological needs and the manner in which they do so will determine the extent to which the child develops trust or mistrust in the surrounding world and the people in it. Those children who develop a sense of trust will acquire the virtue of hope.

Stage 2: Early childhood. Erikson characterized the psychosocial conflict during this stage as autonomy versus shame and doubt. The adaptive emergence from this stage produces the psychological strength of will. The response of the child's caregivers, such as parents, to the child's growing abilities and need to do things for himself or herself will determine whether the child will demonstrate self-sufficiency or self-doubt.

Stage 3: Play age. The psychosocial crisis presented during this stage of development is that of initiative versus guilt. Children who are provided with the opportunity to initiate motor and intellectual skills will acquire the psychological strength or virtue of purpose. The ability to play, which is acquired during this stage, will become the basis in later years for a sense of humor. Those who are not provided with such supportive opportunities will develop a sense of guilt.

Stage 4: School age. This period of development is marked by a conflict between industry and inferiority. An adaptive child learns to love to learn and to play in a manner consistent with what Erikson has called the "ethos of production" (Erikson, 1997, p. 75) and develops a sense of competence. Maladaptation is characterized by excessive competition or the development of a sense of inferiority.

Stage 5. Adolescence. Adolescence reflects the conflict between identity and role confusion. During this stage of development the individual must selectively integrate experiences of childhood and the various images that the individual may have of himself or herself. Individuals must engage in a certain amount of role repudiation in order to accomplish this integration of self-development; some roles may actually jeopardize the synthesis of the individual's identity and must therefore be discarded. Successful integration will yield the psychological strength or virtue of fidelity, which is related to both infantile trust and adult faith. In contrast, individuals who do not pass through this stage of development may engage in more global role repudiation, potentially leading to systematic defiance or the development of a negative identity consisting of socially unacceptable behaviors and traits.

Stage 6. Young adulthood. During young adulthood, individuals must develop the capacity to become intimate with and care about others. The challenge is to be able to commit oneself in a relationship that may require compromise and sacrifice. The antithesis to this intimacy is isolation, which may be associated with a fear of losing one's identity in a relationship. Individuals who successfully resolve this conflict acquire the ability to love and exhibit healthy patterns of cooperation and competition in their relations with others.

Stage 7. Adulthood. The seventh stage reflects the crisis of generativity versus self-absorption and stagnation. Generativity encompasses procreativity, productivity, and creativity, ushering in new beings (children) as well as new ideas and products. In contrast, those who stagnate remain focused on their own wants and desires, resulting in what Erikson has called "generative frustration" (Erikson, 1997, p. 68). The virtue or strength that is derived from successful resolution of this conflict is "care," meaning a broader commitment to care for persons, products, and ideas. The virtue or strength of care may extend to the idea of universal care, such as care for the welfare of all children.

Stage 8. Old age. Erikson hypothesized that the final stage of life is characterized by the conflict between integrity and despair (Erikson, 1997). During this stage, the individual will look back over his or her life. They may view their life as having been satisfying and meaningful (integrity) or as deeply unsatisfying (despair). The former response implies an acceptance of death and a philosophical perspective, while the latter suggests a fear of death and "the feeling that time is now short, too short for the attempt to start another life and to try out alternate roads . . ." (Erikson, 1951, p. 269). Those who are able to pass through this stage successfully will have developed wisdom.

Stage 9. Gerotranscendence. Erikson's original stage model of psychosocial development comprised only eight stages of development. However, a ninth stage was later added to this model to reflect the conflict that arises during the very latest years of life (Erikson, 1997).

This ninth stage of development, corresponding to the 80s and 90s in life, is often characterized by a pervasive sense of loss—of one's physical senses, such as the ability to hear and to see; of friends and family members who have predeceased the elder; of recognition by others as a source of knowledge and wisdom. Joan Erikson (1997, p. 114) has characterized the dilemma facing elders at this stage of their lives:

> [O]ur society does not truly know how to integrate elders into its primary patterns or conventions or into its vital functioning. Rather than be included, aged individuals are often ostracized, neglected, and overlooked; elders are seen no longer as bearers of wisdom but as embodiments of shame.

Consequently, the stage of gerotranscendence may reflect a conflict between a sense of deepening despair associated with the hurdles, burdens, and losses of older age and basic trust and hope, which gives rise to continued reason for living.

Other scholars have expanded on Erikson's concepts. As an example, John Kotre (1984, p. 10) defined generativity as "a desire to invest one's substance in forms of life and work that will outlive the self." He hypothesized that there exist four major types of generativity. These include (1) the biological type, which focuses on the bearing and nursing of offspring; (2) the parental type, which emphasizes the nurturing and disciplining of offspring and their initiation into family traditions; (3) the technical type, involving the transmission of knowledge and skills to successors; and (4) the cultural type, which deals with the creation, renovation, and conservation of a symbol system and its transmittal to successors.

However, there has also been significant disagreement about the basic premise underlying Erikson's model, that individuals necessarily pass through stages and that these stages occur in lockstep or sequential fashion. These criticisms have included the rigidity and deterministic nature of a stage model itself; the failure to delineate clear beginnings and endpoints of each stage; the interpretation of individuals' deviations from the enumerated stages as signifying maladjustment; and the failure to consider the social and historical context of individuals' development and the corresponding need to consider the hypothesized stages of life cycle development in the specific social and historical context (Falicov, 1984; Peck, 1968; Weiland, 1992).

Various scholars have proposed alternative models for the examination of adult growth and development. For instance, McCrae and Costa (1990, 1997) have focused their work on building an understanding of individual adaptation as a function of the interaction between the individual's personality and the environment. They developed a five-factor model of personality, arguing that all individuals possess each of the traits in varying degrees and that the more of a trait that a person possesses, the more likely he or she will be to evidence behaviors generally associated with such traits. This five-factor model encompassed (1) neuroticism, meaning the likelihood that the individual will experience unpleasant emotions and how they react to them; (2) extraversion, or the extent to which the individual prefers social interaction and activity; (3) openness, or the degree to which the individual is receptive to new ideas and experiences; (4) agreeableness, referring to the individual's level of compassion and motivation to avoid conflict, among other qualities; and (5) conscientiousness, meaning the extent to which the individual is or is not ambitious and organized, in addition to related qualities (McCrae & Costa, 1990, 1997).

Despite the criticisms of Erikson's model of psychosocial development, the model itself can serve as a metaphor. The metaphor of the ladder can be used to help clients assess where they are in their own growth and develop their vision for the subsequent stages of their lives. The counselor or therapist can also use the metaphor to assess the client's growth during the course of therapy. The universality of the ladder as a symbol further facilitates its use as a metaphor.

THE METAPHOR OF THE LADDER

The ladder has been used as a symbol by groups holding widely diverse beliefs. In the Old Testament, we are told the story of Jacob and the ladder:

> He [Jacob] had a dream in which he saw a ladder resting on the earth, with its top reaching to heaven, and the angels of God were ascending and descending on it. There above it stood the Lord, and he said: "I am the God of your father Abraham and the God of Isaac. I will give you and your descendants the land on which you are lying. Your descendants will be like the dust of the earth, and you will spread out to the west and to the east, to the north and to the south. All peoples on earth shall be blessed through you and your offspring (Genesis 28:12–14).

In this context, we see that the ladder symbolizes a connection linking heaven to earth (Cirlot, 2002) and God to man.

The Qur'an similarly uses the ladder as a symbol of the link between Heaven and Earth, between man and God. Sûrah 6:35 states:

> And if their aversion is grievous unto thee, then, if thou canst, seek a way down into the earth or a ladder unto the sky that thou mayst bring unto them a portent (to convince them all!)—if Allah willed, He could have brought them all together to the guidance—So be not thou among the foolish ones.

Albrecht Dürer's drawing titled "Melencolia I," executed in 1514, used the symbolism of the ladder to depict this connection between Heaven and Earth. There, each of the ladder's seven rungs symbolized one of the seven basic metals relied upon by alchemy—gold, silver, mercury, copper, lead, tin, and iron (Kruger, 1999). The soul was to accomplish its ascent to Heaven one step at a time. Not surprisingly, then, the ladder has come to represent, as well, both the various levels of consciousness that exist between Man and his divine self and the achievement of wholeness or unity (Hamilton-Parker, 1999). Descent from the ladder has come to mean an attempt to escape from one's spiritual responsibilities.

The Jewish philosopher Maimonides, who was born in Córdoba, Spain, in 1135 and who later fled to Egypt following the invasion of Spain by fundamentalist Muslims from Morocco, used the ladder and its steps to symbolize the various levels of charitable giving. The lowest rung represented somewhat grudging giving by a known donor to a known recipient, potentially resulting in a sense of shame, embarrassment, and obligation on the part of the recipient. In contrast, the highest rung of this ladder of charity was said to consist of giving in a manner designed to develop self-sufficiency (Salamon, 2003).

USING THE METAPHOR

Clients may wish to use the metaphor in various ways apart from such an assessment of their growth. They may, for instance, visualize the various rungs of the ladder as corresponding to critical events or turning points in their own lives, when they had to make major decisions or when external events changed the course of their lives.

You may remember Joseph, who, as explained in other chapters, had been diagnosed with dysthymia and presented with numerous issues ranging from a dysfunctional family life and history of childhood sexual abuse to questions about his own sexual identity to neighborhood violence. Joseph used the metaphor of the ladder to look at his personal situation in the context of his larger environment. He put where he had been at the very lowest rung of the ladder: unemployed, abusing alcohol and marijuana, engaging in anonymous sexual encounters with multiple partners. As he could see himself making progress towards his goals, he gradually moved himself up the various rungs of the ladder: up one step for having completed his GED, up another step for enrolling in college, successfully completing a few courses, and obtaining and keeping steady employment. At the very highest rung of the ladder, Joseph said, was having a stable job, a life that was good and meaningful, and good housing. Joseph's use of the ladder metaphor in this manner was actually reminiscent of Maslow's hierarchy of needs.

At one point in time, Joseph lent his newly purchased previously-owned car to a friend. Joseph had let the insurance on the car lapse because he did not have money for the premium, having spent that money on a new cell phone and new clothing. The friend had a car accident, leaving the car in an undrivable condition and requiring thousands of dollars in repairs, the value of which was more than Joseph continued to owe on the car. Joseph was surprised when the friend refused to contribute to the cost of the car repairs. Joseph moved himself back down the ladder by two rungs for having neglected his budget and having made poor decisions regarding the use of his car and his selection of friends.

Geoffrey used the metaphor of the ladder in much the same way as Joseph did. Geoffrey, it was explained earlier, was suffering from acute symptoms of schizophrenia and had gone to live with his father and his father's wife in a highly conservative rural area of his state. In this setting, Geoffrey was incessantly bombarded with warnings about his destined place in hell as a result of his homosexuality. In addition, he felt infantilized as his father refused either to relinquish control over the management of Geoffrey's finances, even after Geoffrey's mental health had improved significantly, or to permit any of Geoffrey's friends to visit with him.

In using the ladder metaphor, Geoffrey identified the bottom rung as representing him at the worst point of his mental illness, when he was hearing multiple unidentified voices that continuously criticized his behavior as foolish and Geoffrey as stupid and a failure; had lost his job; had had to claim bankruptcy because of his loss of income from employment and consequent inability to pay his debts; and had lost all of his savings, which his father had unilaterally claimed as compensation for having taken him in. Geoffrey gradually moved up the rungs of the ladder that he constructed: first, his relocation to his own apartment in a building for severely mentally ill persons in transition; second, obtaining part-time contract employment while living in his own apartment and learning how to use a laptop computer; third, moving out of the rural area into a larger city and assuming full-time employment and stable housing; fourth, maintaining everything he had achieved at the previous rung, being able to establish a savings account, and reconnecting with friends he had had prior to the onset of his illness symptoms.

In contrast to the manner in which both Joseph and Geoffrey used the ladder metaphor as both measures of their ability to move out of their environments and as a way of identifying their goals and the progress that they were making in achieving them, Wally's use of the ladder metaphor more closely reflected Erikson's depiction of life as a succession of stages. Wally's situation, discussed in greater detail in Chapter 9, was in his mid-60s, continuing with his professional work on a part-time basis, and spending the greater portion of his days caring for his wife, who had been diagnosed with early-onset Alzheimer's disease. Perhaps prompted in part by his wife's deteriorating mental and physical health and feeling the need to maintain an emotional connection with her as long as possible before her recognition of him ceased entirely, Wally began the process of looking back on his life to review the years that he had spent with his wife, their trials and joys raising their children, their more private moments together, and his individual and professional successes. He viewed his life as having been both meaningful and productive and used his past accomplishments and pleasures as the basis to project his future during the next phase of his life, after his beloved wife Crystal was no longer present.

REFERENCES

Cirlot, J. E. (2002). *A dictionary of symbols* (2nd ed.). Mineola, NY: Dover Publications.

Erikson, E. (1951). *Childhood and society.* New York: W. W. Norton & Company.

Erikson, E. (1964). *Insight and responsibility.* New York: W. W. Norton & Company.

Erikson, E. (1997). *The life cycle completed (extended version).* New York: W. W. Norton & Company.

Falicov, C. (1984). Commentary: Focus on stages. *Family Process, 23,* 329–334.

Hamilton-Parker, C. (1999). *The hidden meaning of dreams.* New York: Sterling Publishing Co., Inc.

Kotre, J. (1984). *Outliving the self: Generativity and the interpretation of lives.* Baltimore, Maryland: Johns Hopkins University Press.

Kruger, A. (1999). *ArtBook Dürer.* London: Dorling Kindersley Publishing, Inc.

McCrae, R. R., & Costa, P. T., Jr. (1990). *Personality in adulthood.* New York: Guilford Press.

McCrae, R. R., & Costa, P. T., Jr. (1997). Personality trait structure as a human universal. *American Psychologist, 52,* 509–516.

Peck, R. (1968). Psychological developments in the second half of life. In B. Neugarten (Ed.), *Middle age and aging* (pp. 88–92). Chicago: University of Chicago Press.

Salamon, J. (2003). *Rambam's ladder: A meditation on generosity and why it is necessary to give.* New York: Workman Publishing.

Weiland, S. (1993). Erik Erikson: Ages, stages, and stories. *Generations, 17,* 17–22.

SUGGESTIONS FOR FURTHER READING

Adult Development

Levinson, D. (1978). *The seasons of a man's life.* New York: Ballantine Books.

Mercer, R. T., Nichols, E. G., & Doyle, G. C. (1989). *Transitions in a woman's life: Major life events in developmental context.* New York: Springer.

Aging, Creativity, and Productivity

Lehman, H. C. (1953). *Age and achievement.* Princeton, NJ: Princeton University Press.

Simonton, D. K. (1990). Creativity and wisdom in aging. In J. E. Birren & K. W. Schaie (Eds.), *Handbook of the psychology of aging* (3rd ed., pp. 320–329). San Diego, CA: Academic Press.

Working with Older Adults

Frazer, D. W., & Jongsma, A. E., Jr. (1999). *The older adult psychotherapy treatment planner.* New York: John Wiley & Sons, Inc.

Knight, B. G. (2004). *Psychotherapy with older adults.* Thousand Oaks, CA: Sage.

CHAPTER 7

Follow The Yellow Brick Road:

The Quest for the Unknown Self

THE UNKNOWN SELF

Carl Jung hypothesized that each individual is on a quest for a sense of meaning and the achievement of personal integration and a sense of wholeness (Jung, 1938). He called this integration of the self "individuation." This integration of oneself, Jung postulated, requires that the individual both recognize and own those parts of himself or herself that could be considered "lesser than." Jung explained that

> whoever looks into the mirror of the water will see first of all his own face. Whoever goes to himself risks a confrontation with himself. The mirror does not flatter, it faithfully shows whatever looks into it; namely, the face we never show to the world because we cover it with the *persona*, the mask of the actor (Jung, *Archetypes of the collective unconscious*, quoted in Staub de Laszlo, 1993, p. 381).

Jung called this unknown portion of the self the "shadow." He noted the difficulty inherent in knowing one's shadow:

> The shadow is a living part of the personality and therefore wants to live with it in some form. It cannot be argued out of existence or rationalized into harmlessness. This problem is exceedingly difficult, because it not only challenges the whole man, but reminds him at the same time of his helplessness and ineffectuality. Strong natures—or should one rather call them weak?—do not like to be reminded of this, but prefer to think of themselves as heroes who are beyond good and evil . . . (Jung, *Archetypes of the collective unconscious*, quoted in Staub de Laszlo, 1993, p. 381).

The individual without a shadow, Jung claimed, is the individual who believes that he consists of only what he wishes to know about himself (Jung, 1969). Jung believed that one's knowledge of one's own shadow, or dark side of one's personality, would come about naturally in the course of reasonably comprehensive therapy (Jung, *The religious and psychological problems of alchemy,* in Staub de Laszlo, 1993).

Although Jung conceived of the shadow as an unwelcome or displeasing quality that might be difficult to acknowledge, the shadow might just as well comprise qualities that could be thought of as "good," but that the individual is unable or unwilling to acknowledge because those "good" qualities are at odds with the story that has been told about the individual by others and that he or she has accepted. The metaphor of *The Wizard of Oz* or the "yellow brick road" is a powerful tool to discover both qualities that could be considered positive and those that might be considered negative. In using this metaphor with clients, I ask what knowledge about themselves would await them. What part of themselves have they been unable to acknowledge in order to attain wholeness?

THE METAPHOR OF *THE WIZARD OF OZ*

You may remember the story of *The Wizard of Oz* (Baum, 1999). Although there are many differences between the original novel by Baum and the MGM movie production based on that story, the basic plot is the same. Dorothy and her family, who are living in Kansas, must seek shelter from a tornado. Dorothy's aunt and uncle, with whom she is living, safely reach the storm shelter in time to escape the tornado. Dorothy, however, receives a blow to her head. She and her faithful dog Toto find themselves in the Land of Oz, populated by the Munchkins and terrorized by the Wicked Witch of the East. Dorothy's house falls on the Wicked Witch, resulting in her death, at which the Munchkins rejoice. Desperately wishing to return home, she is advised to seek out the Wizard in the Emerald City, who will best be able to advise her. Glinda, the Good Witch, uses her powers to place the slippers once worn by the now-deceased witch on Dorothy's feet, advising her not to remove them.

En route to the Emerald City, Dorothy encounters the Scarecrow, who has no brain; the Tin Man, who lacks a heart; and the Lion, who is without courage. They accompany Dorothy on her journey to find the Wizard, helping each other to overcome the obstacles and difficulties placed in their path by the Wicked Witch of the West. Later, they must confront the Wicked Witch directly in order to obtain her broom, which the Wizard has demanded as a precondition to his granting of their requests. Finally, they return to the Emerald City, only to find that the Wizard is actually a fraud and cannot bestow on them the qualities that they have been seeking. They each find in themselves what it is that they were searching for elsewhere: a brain for Scarecrow, a heart for Tin Man, and courage for Lion. Dorothy needs only to tap the heels of the slippers together and acknowledge that "There's no place like home" to find that she is there and never really left those who love her.

USING THE METAPHOR

Because individuals of all ages are familiar with the story of *The Wizard of Oz*, and the story itself is so powerful, I have been able to use it as a metaphor in my work with adults of all ages. I use the story of *The Wizard of Oz* as a tool to help clients discover who they would find that they really are if they were to follow The Yellow Brick Road.

Geoffrey, who, as you may remember from previous chapters, had been diagnosed with schizophrenia, related that his father and siblings had told him throughout his life, "You don't know anything. Get a clue." He grew up believing that he could not trust his understandings or perceptions. That belief was reinforced even further with the diagnosis of schizophrenia, which seemingly validated the judgment of his father, brother, and sister. I did not use the metaphor of the Yellow Brick Road with Geoffrey until well into our relationship, so that he would have the opportunity to reflect back and decipher something positive that he had learned through the many sessions that we had had. When I asked him what quality he believed he lacked that he discovered he actually possesses, he responded, "My insight. I am much more insightful about myself and others and in general than I thought." His observation was, indeed, accurate. Despite his illness, he was often attuned to the underlying dynamics and motivations of people and situations that he encountered.

Joseph, who had been diagnosed with dysthymia, welcomed the opportunity to "follow the yellow brick road." He was immediately able to identify qualities that he believed he lacked, to a large degree based on what others had told him about himself. However, he was not able to say which ones he actually possessed of those he believed were missing. As part of this exercise, I asked Joseph to make a list on a daily basis for one week of everything he did that he thought was good, to be discussed at our subsequent session.

Joseph came to the next session beaming. He had made a list of the many things that he did for others during the previous week and of things that he did that he felt good about. Using this list, he recited the qualities that he had found that he actually possessed.

Joseph's grandmother, with whom he lived as a child and young adult, had consistently reprimanded him for his selfishness towards others.

Consequently, Joseph grew up believing that he was inconsiderate of others and their needs and attentive only to his own desires. By making the list as he went down "the yellow brick road" that week, he discovered that he actually did quite a large number of favors for individuals that he cared about, including his grandmother, and that in many ways he was quite generous with his time and his limited amount of cash.

Joseph felt that his grandmother had always disparaged his attempts to learn and to test out newly learned skills, telling him, "You ain't never gonna amount to nothin.' You ain't nothin' and you never gonna be nothin'." Joseph had believed to his core that he was a failure and could never succeed at anything. As he went "down the yellow brick road" for one week, he found that he kept his appointments, showed up to his college classes on time, arrived at his job in a timely manner, dressed appropriately for various occasions, and was seen as a role model by many of the youth who attended a community center where he volunteered. He drove his car without incident, did favors for his friends, and received praise for the hard work he did in his counseling session. Joseph concluded, after reciting his list, "I am something. I'm actually slightly proud of myself."

George's situation illustrates how the metaphor can be used to help individuals identify and come to terms with those parts of themselves that they think might be "bad." George was a young man in late adolescence who had grown up in an inner city neighborhood. He had been in trouble many times because, he explained, he "hung with the wrong crowd." He had a long history of gang involvement, fights, and drug use. As he said, he had done things he wasn't very proud of.

It took George over a year to go down the Yellow Brick Road to accept the fact of his homosexuality, which members of his family and community would consider a sin. George was ultimately able to recognize that the violence that he had previously directed outwards towards others was the externalization of the anger and fear that he felt towards himself and a mechanism by which to avoid recognizing and addressing his sexual orientation. Ultimately, George located a community center that welcomed individuals regardless of their sexual orientation, met people who were comfortable with their "gayness" and, through counseling and extended interaction with positive role models, was able to accept his own sexuality.

Sometimes, asking individuals to identify their "missing" negative quality as they proceed down the Yellow Brick Road may be unsuccessful; they may be unwilling to identify or acknowledge out loud those qualities that may be seen by themselves or others as negative or "bad." In such situations, I have continued to utilize the metaphor of The Wizard of Oz, but with variations on the theme. One such variation is to suggest that the Wizard was ultimately found to be a fraud because he was unable to help Dorothy and her friends find their desired qualities; they already possessed them and had only to recognize them in themselves. Using this observation as the foundation, I might ask "What about yourself are you afraid that people might realize isn't real? What would happen?"

Sometimes clients' answers may not be what you might expect. Once, when I was conducting a group session with men only, one of the men gulped slowly before speaking. Andrew, a young man in his mid-20s, began to talk about a previous romantic relationship that he had been involved in with another man. Andrew often gave others the impression that he was self-sufficient, independent, and self-knowledgeable. His greatest fear had been that people would discover that his previous partner had physically abused him, his emotional vulnerability, and the attending shame that had prevented him from seeking the counseling and support services that he had so desperately needed at that time. Other participants in the group expressed their sympathy and support. Andrew's courageous disclosure gave several other men the courage to similarly disclose their pasts as either victims of abuse or abusers themselves, and the shame and guilt that they lived with knowing what they had done to people whom they had professed to love.

Even with these variations of the metaphor, some clients may continue to experience difficulty acknowledging those parts of themselves that they don't like or with which they are uncomfortable. However, integration will never truly be possible unless and until one is able to recognize the component parts of oneself. Consequently, it is important to find a strategy or mechanism that will facilitate the client's recognition of himself or herself. In such situations, I have suggested to clients that they identify either a character in *The Wizard of Oz* or a fairy tale or storybook character who seems to reflect who the clients are and discuss how they and the character are similar. We can then use their identified character as a starting point to explore what Jung would call the client's shadow.

The following is an excerpt from a group session attended by seven individuals, each of whom had received a diagnosis of bipolar disorder. Group participants had not been able, in general, to identify with any character of *The Wizard of Oz*, but they quickly latched onto the idea of themselves as a fairy tale or fantasy character.

EDGAR: At first I thought Jack and the Beanstalk, but then I thought Pinocchio. Because my whole life has been a lie. Not objectively, but in my head. It was all lies. Work was going great, my relationships were great. Not really, but in my head. Then it all fell apart. It was easier to lie. Now it's all black and white, you either lie or tell the truth, no gray, nothing in between. People either want you to lie or tell the truth and when you tell the truth, they get angry. It's like Pinocchio. He turns into a real boy when he tells the truth but it is painful.

PAUL: I feel like Dr. Jekyll and Mr. Hyde. It's seductive, raw, senseless. It's hard to give up.

SL: What do you mean by seductive?

PAUL: You do what you want. I don't have much guilt, I never have. You just say and do what you want. But I have children. My children are important to me and I wouldn't want to leave them like that. But it's hard. It feels like you're wading in water way up to your neck and you have to push through. I feel so angry. Sometimes, not to offend anyone, but I imagine I have a terminal illness and I have six months to live. I'd just go out and, bang, knock off a few people. A lot of people deserve to be knocked off.

DENNIS: I know what you mean. Sometimes I think about having a terminal illness and living only six months but then I could go out and take care of everything, do everything I want and then be done, just finish life.

SL: Would that give you more control?

DENNIS: You'd know.

ALICE: I feel like Elfaba. The play *Wicked*, what happened before *The Wizard of Oz*. Glinda and Elfaba were friends and everyone loved Glinda. Elfaba was different, you can see, and she told the truth. She didn't lie. And people cast her out and she stopped trying, she became hateful. And that's what I feel like.

SL: So you feel like you are hateful?

ALICE: Every morning I go to work. I work at a day care. I work with the babies, they are so wonderful. You say anything to them and they smile at you. You can say, oh, look at your toes for 45 minutes and they laugh and smile. And then the staff, they say why aren't you fixed yet? Your mother [in the hospital] will be fine. Why can't you be happy? I didn't know there was a time limit on being sad.

EDGAR: They said that? "Why can't you be fixed?"

ALICE: That's what they said.

EDGAR: I would be angry, too.

ALICE: So I don't care. I do everything to please everyone else, my boss, my mother. And then I get angry. I try to tell the truth and then I feel like I am punished for telling the truth. I let people in traffic and in southern Ohio they'll wave and say thank you, but not here.

EDGAR: That gets to me, too.

BRENDA: I know what you mean.

EDGAR: You need to make a list. You need to make a list with three columns, one column for what makes you happy and one column for what works now, what helps you get through things. That way you can look at the list and see what helps you get through things.

PAUL: It seems to me that you're way ahead of the game. You know what your issues are. I hear you talk about the babies and I am jealous. That sounds beautiful.

ALICE: I love it with them.

BRENDA: Lamb Chop.

SL: Like Sheri Lewis?

BRENDA: Yes.

SL: Why Lamb Chop?

BRENDA: I don't know.

SL: What do you like about Lamb Chop?

BRENDA: She's sweet and smiles and people like her.

SL: Is that what you're like?

BRENDA: No, I'm argumentative. I challenge everything. Not with my closest friends, but with everyone else, I have to argue.

SL: Is that what you want to be?

BRENDA: It's not good for relationships. Sometimes I catch myself and then I try to calm down and say to myself, why are you doing this, you're not happy. I try to stop myself and enjoy myself. I try to be pleasant with people, to say things differently.

DARLA: I feel like Wile E. Coyote. I'm always chasing my sanity. All my life, chasing the sanity and then just when you think you have it, something blows up. No matter what I do, I can't control it. There's an R & B [rhythm and blues] song, I like R & B, that says, that has a line, "The hunter gets captured by the game," on Motown. I'm always hunting my sanity. All the world's a stage and each one plays a part. I'm full of lines today. I'm just trying to find my space in life. I've lost me, my total personality. I believe in God and Satan and heaven and hell and God put demons on this earth. Like the people I work with. They're evil. . . .

KATRINA: In the movie *Shrek*, Princess Fiona was always preoccupied with her appearance and that's the way I've been my whole life, so you don't really know who you are inside at your core.

SL: Who are you at your core?

KATRINA: I don't know. I'm trying to find out. My memory isn't good. I don't remember, maybe from being ill.

It is important to note how various clients used the idea of this metaphor. Some relied on it to reflect who they are now and why they are unhappy with this state of being, while others chose a character that reflected who or what they would like to be. In either instance, the client's selection of character and observations about that character suggest what part the client believes is missing. It affords the therapist the opportunity to explore with the client on an individual basis those qualities that the client would like to have, the extent to which that image is realistic, and the nature of those qualities that the client believes that he or she lacks. For instance, in response to Brenda's wish to be more like Lamb Chop, the therapist might explore what qualities that Lamb Chop has are desirable to the client; how often Brenda might like to be like that; whether it is realistic to reflect those qualities, such as being "nice" and "sweet," in all situations; and whether there exist alternative approaches to integrate the desired qualities with Brenda's personality and existing strengths.

Because group members had not previously been in groups that utilized this technique, I asked them to comment on what they thought or felt about the exercise. Their responses were generally favorable.

KATRINA: Good. No one ever made us look at who we are and think about what we want to be.

ALICE: I have a hard time expressing myself and saying what I want and feel. I am always saying things to please people. It was good to be able to say what I feel. I felt, I felt connected.

PAUL: You're not numb, you can express yourself.

DARLA: This was really good. I didn't know how I was feeling. It was good to get it out.

EDGAR: I really liked this. It finally made sense to me and helped me put it together . . . this made me think.

PAUL: It was good. It is difficult being so vulnerable, opening yourself up like this in a group. It was good. I learned a lot.

DENNIS: It was good. All the things here helped me.

DARLA: I need validation. I have a right to be angry. Don't I have a right to be angry?

ALICE: You do. It's okay to be angry. You have a right.

Characters from *The Wizard of Oz* and other stories can also be used to help clients explore parts of themselves and their relations with others. For instance, you might ask clients to identify that part of themselves that is most like Glinda the Good Witch, or that is most like the Wicked Witch of the West. Alternatively, they may identify someone in their family or their constellation of friends and coworkers as the Wicked Witch with whom they must do battle. You can then explore with them the dynamics of the situation, what they bring to the conflict, and the strategies (weapons) that they might bring to bear to ameliorate or eliminate the conflict.

As with other metaphors, the metaphor of *The Wizard of Oz* can be used at various points in time over the course of a longer-term therapeutic relationship. As individuals grow in their awareness of themselves, they may continue to discover different aspects of their shadow, qualities that they had heretofore been unable or unwilling to see. The character that they select as reflective of who they are, whether it is a positive or negative image, may provide clues as to the direction and extent of their personal growth during the course of therapy. As such, the metaphor serves as both an indication of where they are in their quest for individuation and how far they have journeyed.

Because the metaphor of *The Wizard of Oz* is deeply rooted in American culture, it may not be helpful to individuals whose heritage and/or affinity lies with other cultures, such as newly immigrated individuals and non-English speakers. When working with such clients on an individual basis or in the context of a group, it is advisable to use the metaphor of a fantasy or mythical figure. When group members have diverse cultural backgrounds and they choose characters that are unfamiliar to the other group members, it will be helpful to both the individual client and the other group members to have the client explain his or her particular selection; that explanation can then be used as the basis to explore with clients the question of who they believe they are now or what qualities they would like to develop.

REFERENCES

Baum, L. F. (1999). *The wizard of Oz*. New York: Simon & Schuster.

Jung, C. G. (1938). *Psychology and religion*. New Haven, CT: Yale University Press.

Jung, C.G. (1969). *The nature of the psyche* (Trans. R. F. C. Hull). Princeton, NJ: Princeton University Press.

Staub de Laszlo, V. (Ed.). (1993). *The basic writings of C.G. Jung*. New York: Random House, Inc.

SUGGESTIONS FOR FURTHER READING

Cross-cultural Counseling and Storytelling

Costantino, G., Malgady, R. G., & Rogler, L. H. (1986). Cuento therapy: A culturally sensitive modality for Puerto Rican children. *Journal of Consulting and Clinical Psychology, 54,* 639–645.

Malgady, R. G., Rogler, L. H., & Costantino, G. (1990). Hero/heroine modeling for Puerto Rican adolescents: A preventive mental health intervention. *Journal of Consulting and Clinical Psychology, 58,* 469–474.

Fairy Tales, Fantasy, and Therapy

Bettelheim, B. (1977). *The use of enchantment: The importance and meaning of fairy tales.* New York: Vintage.

Gardner, R. (1981). *Therapeutic communication with children: The mutual storytelling technique.* New York: Science House.

Individuation and Unity

Assagioli, R. (1965). *Psychosynthesis: A collection of basic writings.* New York: Penguin Press.

Rowan, J. (1993). *The transpersonal: Psychotherapy and counseling.* London: Routledge Press.

CHAPTER 8

Stone Soup:

Altruism for Health

THE IMPORTANCE OF GIVING TO OTHERS

All of the world's religions concur that giving to others is virtuous (Neusner & Chilton, 2005). In Judaism, for example, self-motivated acts of kindness are believed to be worthy of divine reward, eliciting God's empathy, just as sinful acts bring about His punishment (Neusner & Avery-Peck, 2005). Proverbs 11:16 tells us, "A kindhearted woman gains respect, but ruthless men gain only wealth," while Proverbs 11:17 advises, "A kind man benefits himself, but a cruel man brings trouble on himself." Proverbs 11:25 counsels, "A generous man will prosper; he who refreshes others will himself be refreshed."

In Christianity, the story in John's Gospel of Jesus washing the feet of his disciples illustrates the nature and importance of giving and doing for others:

> He said to them. Do you know what I have done for you? You call me teacher and lord, and you say well; I am. If, then, I—lord and teacher—washed your feet, you also ought to wash one another's feet. For I have given you an example, so that just as I have done to you, so you also might do. Truly, truly I say to you, a servant is not greater than his lord, nor an apostle greater than the one who sent him. If you know these things, you are blessed if you do them.

We are told in Galatians 6:9, as well, that those who act for the benefit of others will be rewarded: "Let us not become weary in doing good, for at the proper time we will reap a harvest if we do not give up."

Buddhism teaches that suffering is universal; compassion is the proper response to this reality (Lewis, 2005). A biography of the Buddha tells us:

Those who in charity renounce their wealth
Cleanse away avarice and attachment.
Giving in compassion and respect,
They drive away envy, hatred, and pride (Robinson, 1954, p. 11).

The giving is believed to bring benefit to the giver through the law of karma, the universal law that every action brings about a just moral retributive action (Schumann, 1973; Smith, 1991).

Buddhism has also recognized that the ability to give to others varies depending upon one's circumstances in life. Mahayana Buddhism teaches:

Good Son, there are three fundamentals to all kinds of giving: (1) giving compassionately to the poor, (2) giving to foes without seeking rewards, and (3) giving joyfully and respectfully to the virtuous. . . . If one can teach others before giving them material things, one is called a great giver . . . . if a wise person is wealthy, he should give like that. If he is not wealthy, he should teach other wealthy people to practice giving. . . . If he is poor and has nothing to give, he should recite curative mantras, give inexpensive medicines to the needy, sincerely take care of the ill for recuperation, and exhort the rich to provide medicines; if he knows medical remedies . . . he should provide treatment according to the diagnosis . . . (Shih, 1994, ch. 19).

Similar to Buddhism, Islam recognizes that giving benefits the giver as well as the recipient. The Qur'an states:

There are others who acknowledge their misdeeds and their mixing of good deed with bad. Perhaps God will forgive them, for God is forgiving and merciful. Accept from their wealth alms (*sadaqh*) with which you may purify them and make them prosper (9:102–3, quoted in Homerin, 2005, p. 71).

Philosophers and poets also tell us of the value of doing good for others. Tulsidas, a 16th century Hindu poet, wrote,

This and this alone is true religion—to serve others. This is sin above all other sin—to harm others. In service to others is happiness. In selfishness is misery and pain (Post, 2008, p. 18).

Shantideva, a ninth-century sage, advised, "All the joy the world contains has come through wishing the happiness of others" (Post, 2008, p. 19).

Even Aesop's fables (1947) speak of the value of doing good for others. Aesop tells us the story of the lion and the mouse. The mouse, crossing the path of the lion, pleads with him to spare his life, promising to remember this act of kindness and to repay it should the opportunity to do so ever arise. The lion, disbelieving that he would ever need the help of the small mouse, releases him nevertheless. Not long afterwards, the lion is caught in a net that was set out by hunters to trap him. The mouse nibbled at the ropes with his teeth until the lion was freed. The moral of the story, we are told, is that "No act of kindness, no matter how small, is ever wasted" (Aesop, 1947, p. 138).

In addition to receiving spiritual and material benefits by giving to others, givers may also improve their own physical health through the act of giving. Social interest, reflecting the ability to value the interests and welfare of others even in the absence of personal utility (Crandall, 1981), has been found to be associated with better life adjustment (Crandall & Lehman, 1977) and better physical health status (Zarski, Bubenzer, & West, 1986). The provision of social support to others has been associated with better health (Brown, Consedine, & Magai, 2005). A study of 1,972 California residents found that, even after considering such factors as health habits, physical functioning, and social support, those who volunteered had 44% lower mortality than those who did not (Oman, Thoresen, & McMahon, 1999).

Mental health benefits from giving also may be many and varied. In one study of individuals who helped others, one-half of the participants reported feeling a "helpers' high" when they helped others, and almost one-half reported feeling stronger and more energetic (Luks, 1988). In a study consisting of in-depth interviews with a diverse group of older African American women, the women reported that altruism towards others was an important strategy for their maintenance of good physical and mental health (Unson, Mahoney-Trella, & Chowdhury, 2004). Researchers found from their study of 2,016 members of the Presbyterian Church throughout the United States that, even after considering such factors as age, gender, stressful life events, income, general health, positive and negative religious coping, and asking God for help in healing, individuals who provided help to others had better mental health (Schwartz, Meisenhelder, Ma, & Reed, 2003). The authors of the study concluded that "Helping others is associated with better mental health, above and beyond the benefits of receiving help and other known psychospiritual, stress, and demographic factors" (Schwartz et al., 2003, p. 778).

Research has also demonstrated that social interest in others and helping others is associated with less depression (Crandall, 1975; Krause, Herzog, & Baker, 1992) and less hopelessness (Miller, Denton, & Tobacyk, 1986) and that compassion significantly reduces depression and stress (Steffen & Masters, 2005). Individuals aged 65 and older who volunteer with others actually experience fewer symptoms of depression than those who do not (Musick & Wilson, 2003). Writers have even recognized the value of giving in overcoming feelings of sadness and loneliness. Antoine de Saint-Exupéry wrote, "In giving you are throwing a bridge across the chasm of your solitude" (*The Wisdom of the Sands,* quoted in de Saint-Exupéry, 2002, p. 4).

However, because of the nature of severe mental illness, the concept and act of giving may raise significant issues for some individuals with a severe mental illness. First, they may have difficulty distinguishing between giving that is appropriate and giving that results in their own victimization. Such difficulty may be due to deficits in their ability to process information, which can lead to difficulties in the identification and avoidance of risky situations, as well as deficits in social competence, resulting in turn in a decreased ability to form lasting relationships, refuse unreasonable requests, solve problems effectively, and negotiate risky situations.

Individuals' difficulty identifying appropriate giving may also result from confusion between love and attachment. In referring to attachment as the "near-enemy of love," Kornfield (1988, p. 24) explains:

> It [attachment] masquerades as love. "I love this person, I love this thing," which usually means, "I want to hold it, I want to keep it, I don't want to let it be." This is not love at all; it is attachment and they are different. There is a big difference between love, which allows and honors and appreciates, and attachment, which grasps and holds and aims to possess.

This inability to distinguish between love and attachment may be especially problematic for many individuals with mental illness in the context of romantic and sexual relationships because of their relatively lower levels of self-esteem. "Self-esteem exists along a continuum; individuals are not completely devoid of self-esteem, but neither do individuals have such high levels of self-esteem that they lack the capacity to achieve a higher level of self-esteem" (Branden, 1980, p. 118). Because individuals tend to be attracted to others with similar levels of self-esteem, those with relatively lower levels often select partners who have lower levels of self-esteem themselves. Their insecurities may provide the impetus to engage in behaviors that result in frustration and defeat and ultimately reinforce their feelings of negative self-worth (Branden, 1980). Accordingly, individuals with lower levels of self-esteem may grasp onto unhealthy partner relationships, despite their injurious nature. For individuals with a severe mental illness, this series of events may ultimately result in a heightened risk to them of partner violence (Hatters-Friedman & Loue, 2007) and/or risk of HIV infection (Meade, 2006).

Second, individuals with a mental illness may believe that they have nothing to give to others because of the impact of their mental illness on those around them. They may also be unable to understand the benefits that they could derive themselves from their giving to others. Interactions with family members, coworkers, and others may reinforce these perceptions.

All too often, individuals with a severe mental illness believe, or are made to feel, that they are burdens to their family members, their friends, and their coworkers because of the impact of their illness on those surrounding them. Family members may experience distress from or feel burdened by their ill member's physical complaints, uncooperativeness, and threatening behavior, which may actually be, at least in part, attributable to the mental illness (Grad & Samsbury, 1963; Reinhard & Horwitz, 1995). They may worry about the future and fear for the fate of their loved one (Lefley, 1987; Potasznik & Nelson, 1984; Thomson & Doll, 1982). Parents, in particular, may be emotionally impacted, experiencing self-blame, guilt, or grief because of their child's illness (Loukissa, 1995; MacGregor, 1994; Miller, Dworkin, Ward, & Barone, 1990).

An individual's mental illness may bring about changes in family routines in addition to its emotional impact on other family members. Family members may have to assume household duties that otherwise would have been handled by their ill relative. They may need to provide some level of coordination for the plethora of medical and counseling appointments and may feel some responsibility to ensure that their ill member follows his or her prescribed medication regimen. They may restrict their social activities or availability for employment in order to attend to the needs of their mentally ill family member (Fadden, Bebbington, & Knipers, 1987; Johnson, 1990; Maurin & Boyd, 1990; Reinhard & Horwitz, 1995). This level of participation in the life of a mentally ill family member cannot be shrugged off as "codependence." Frequently, individuals with severe mental illness want to regain and retain their mental health but may be unable to take the necessary steps on their own because of memory difficulties, a lack of understanding of the connection between medications and diminution of symptoms, inertia, or other symptoms of the illness itself.

In situations in which the family member with the mental illness is no longer able to work, even temporarily, other family members may feel the financial strain as a result of lost income to the household and increasing medical and pharmacy bills. The policy of insurers toward restricted mental health care benefits may also result in increased economic strain on the family (Clark, 1994; Grad & Samsbury, 1963).

Coworkers may feel and even express resentment because of the additional duties that they are required to assume during the individual's absence or because of behavior that the individual exhibited as a result of their illness. As an example, an individual with bipolar disorder who is experiencing a manic phase may instigate arguments with coworkers, make inappropriate sexual gestures, or swear at supervisors.

Appropriate giving to others by individuals with a mental illness may be beneficial to the givers as well as to the recipients. Like all individuals, persons with a mental illness have a need to love and to be loved (Alderman & Marshall, 1998). By giving to others, individuals can meet their needs for love and affiliation. And, by recognizing the value of what they bring to their interactions with others, individuals with mental illness may feel increased strength, self-respect, and self-worth (Alderman & Marshall, 1998). These precepts serve as a foundation for the ICCD model (International Center for Clubhouse Development), begun in 1948 by Fountain House in New York City, to provide treatment and socialization opportunities for severely mentally ill persons (American Psychiatric Association, 1999).

THE STORY OF THE STONE SOUP

The story of the stone soup can be used as a vehicle to help individuals think about how they contribute to others, despite their illness. This is an Eastern European folktale, one that has several different versions. One version begins with three soldiers traveling through a strange country on their way home from a war. It is nearly nightfall. They are very hungry and have had nothing to eat for a very long time. They also did not know where they were going to sleep.

As they were walking down the road, they spotted the lights in a village up ahead. They decided to go to the village and ask the people there whether they could sleep in one of their homes, or even a barn, and whether they could have a bite to eat.

When they got to the village, all of the village residents answered that they did not have any food to give them and there was no place for them to sleep. In fact, the villagers had seen them approaching and were afraid of the soldiers. They had hidden all of their food.

The soldiers decided to make stone soup. The villagers had never heard of such a thing! The soldiers asked to borrow a large pot and to use water and to have help to light a fire under the pot. They set the water to boil. Then they asked the villagers to bring them a large stone.

Once the stone was in the pot, the soldiers began to muse out loud about how good it would be if there could be carrots added to the soup but, alas, there were none to be had. One of the villagers suddenly "remembered" that she had carrots and retrieved them to add to the stone soup. This same scenario was repeated with potatoes and meat and cabbage and many other vegetables. Each time one of the soldiers scratched his head and sighed about how wonderful it would be if only they had this or that additional ingredient, one of the villagers would set off to retrieve it and add it to the stone soup.

Finally, the soldiers announced that the soup was ready to be eaten. But, wouldn't it be wonderful if there were bread to accompany the soup and a cold beverage, say, cider or beer, to accompany it all? Sure enough, someone brought bread and someone else contributed cold cider to the meal. The villagers laid out a table with enough places for everyone in the village. After the meal, the villagers invited the soldiers to stay in their homes for the night. After all, without their wisdom, they could not have had such a wonderful feast!

USING THE STORY

There are potentially many "lessons" that can be learned from this story. One such lesson is that everyone has something that they "bring to the table" that helps to nourish both themselves and others. A second teaching of the story is that the whole is always greater than the sum of its parts. The carrots and potatoes and meat and other vegetables are only those things by themselves, but together they make a soup that nourishes the whole village, providing physical nourishment for the body, spiritual nourishment for the soul, and a sense of warmth and belonging.

One group in which I used the story consisted of seven individuals, all diagnosed with depression or bipolar disorder. The three men ranged from 40 to 70 years of age; the women's ages ranged from 38 to 58.

Louis had been suffering from severe depression for an extended period of time. Although he had been attending a cognitive behavioral therapy group for several weeks, I had been told that he rarely spoke and often slept during sessions. Despite his seeming disinterest, Louis became engaged with the group and the telling of his own experiences. He talked about his lengthy battle with depression and the difficulty that he was experiencing in even understanding himself. Ultimately, he concluded that his contribution to others was a teaching of perseverance in the face of seemingly unending obstacles and difficulties.

Other group participants also referred to their illness diagnosis in identifying the qualities that they brought to both the group and to others in their networks. Dustin, a 40-year old man diagnosed with bipolar disorder, spoke of the need for faith in oneself and in others in order to heal and move forward. The group participants told him that he contributed much more than that as a role model and a bearer of wisdom through his life experiences. This positive feedback to Dustin from the group, in addition to his identification of a positive quality that he contributed to the "soup," may have been critical for Dustin, who had consistently seen himself as a burden to others.

Victoria had made multiple suicide attempts throughout her life and had recently been released from the hospital following another such attempt. She suggested that, because she had been suffering with bipolar disorder for most of her adult life, she could contribute a long-term perspective with regard to the illness, its successful management, and pitfalls that individuals might run into during their own struggles with the ups and downs of bipolar disorder. Victoria indicated that she had never before viewed her experiences with her illness as providing any benefit to herself or anyone else. She expressed surprise that her own experiences, both positive and negative, could help others to understand their experiences with their own illness. She became even more amazed when several group members indicated that they valued her as a "teacher" in the group. Victoria had been unaware that others had actually listened to her as she told the story of her efforts to remain mentally healthy despite the repeated resurgence of her symptoms.

Beatrice, who was 57 at the time of this group, was unable to identify any quality that she possessed that could possibly be considered a contribution to this soup. She had been suffering from severe depression for a considerable period of time and was generally silent during group sessions. Others in the group spoke of Beatrice's strength and quiet faith; even though she had to force herself to get out of bed every morning, even though she didn't have the energy to even open her mouth to speak on many days, she forced herself to rise, to wash, to dress, and to attend the group sessions. This, the group suggested, evidenced to them faith in the process of healing and served as an example to them. Beatrice was taken aback by the strength of the group's response to her and her eyes filled with tears.

At the subsequent session with me, group members indicated how important it had been for them to have heard the story of the stone soup and to have been given an opportunity to reflect on its meaning and how it might apply to their own situations. Several of the group members indicated that being able to identify something that they could offer to others had helped them to feel better about themselves.

The therapist can focus on other aspects of the stone soup metaphor depending on the needs of the clients. As an example, consider the situation that confronted the villagers. They were approached by soldiers whose motivations and proclivities were unknown to them. Perhaps they were friendly and merely in need of food and shelter. Or, perhaps this was a ruse that they were using to gain entry into people's homes to pillage and slaughter. We do not know the history of the villagers; perhaps they had been betrayed in the past by persons who professed friendship and caring or who had sought their aid. How can the villagers know whether they can trust these soldiers?

Consider, as well, the plight of the soldiers. They were in need of food and shelter. Should they approach these villagers? Trust them? Perhaps there was a history of which they were unaware and the villagers would seek retribution for those past events through the soldiers. Should the soldiers entrust their lives to these people?

The elucidation of these different perspectives within the story provides an opportunity to explore with clients issues such as vulnerability, trustworthiness, and help-seeking. Clients can use the story to examine the difference between situations in which giving may be appropriate and those in which giving may be harmful to oneself; to identify sources of help for varying needs that they might have and suitable approaches to seeking that help; and to enumerate the type and nature of environmental and interactional cues that can help them assess the safety of a situation and/or the trustworthiness of an individual that they encounter.

REFERENCES

Aesop. (1947). *Aesop's fables.* New York: Grosset & Dunlap. Alderman, T., & Marshall, K. (1998). *Amongst ourselves: A self-help guide to living with dissociative identity disorder.* Oakland, CA: New Harbinger Publications Inc. American Psychiatric Association. (1999). Gold award: The wellspring of the clubhouse model for social and vocational adjustment of persons with serious mental illness. *Psychiatric Services, 50,* 1473–1476.

Branden, N. (1980). *The psychology of romantic love.* Los Angeles: J. P. Tarcher, Inc.

Brown, W. M., Consedine, N. S., & Magai, C. (2005). Altruism relates to health in an ethnically diverse sample of older adults. *The Journal of Gerontology Series B: Psychological and Social Sciences, 60,* 143–152.

Clark, R. E. (1994). Family costs associated with severe mental illness and substance use. *Hospital and Community Psychiatry, 45,* 808–813.

Crandall, J. E. (1975). A scale for social interest. *Journal of Individual Psychology, 31,* 187–195.

Crandall, J. E. (1981). *Theory and measurement of social interest: Empirical tests of Alfred Adler's concepts.* New York: Columbia University Press.

Crandall, J. E., & Lehman, R. E. (1977). Relationship of stressful life events to social interest, locus of control, and psychological adjustment. *Journal of Consulting and Clinical Psychology, 45,* 1208.

de Saint-Exupéry, A. (2002). *A guide for grown-ups: Essential wisdom from the collected works of Antoine de Saint-Exupéry.* San Diego, CA: Harcourt.

Fadden, G., Bebbington, P., & Knipers, A. (1987). The burden of care: The impact of functional psychiatric illness on the patient's family. *British Journal of Psychiatry, 150,* 285–292.

Grad, J., & Samsbury, P. (1963). Mental illness and the family. *Lancet, 1,* 544–547.

Hatters-Friedman, S., & Loue, S. (2007). Incidence and prevalence of intimate partner violence by and against women with severe mental illness. *Journal of Women's Health, 16*(4), 471–480.

Homerin, T. E. (2005). Altruism in Islam. In J. Neusner & B. Chilton (Eds.), *Altruism in world religions* (pp. 67–87). Washington, DC: Georgetown University Press.

Johnson, D. L. (1990). The family's experience of living with mental illness. In H. P. Lefley & D. L. Johnson (Eds.). *Families as allies in the treatment of the mentally ill: New directions for mental health professionals* (pp. 31–64). Arlington, VA: American Psychiatric Press, Inc.

Kornfield, J. (1988). The path of compassion: Spiritual practice and social action. In F. Eppsteiner (Ed.). *The path of compassion: Writings on socially engaged Buddhism* (pp. 24–30). Berkeley, CA: Parallax Press.

Krause, N., Herzog, A. R., & Baker, E. (1992). Providing support to others and well-being in later life. *Journal of Gerontology, 47(5),* 300–311.

Lefley, H. P. (1987). Aging parents as caregivers of mentally ill adult children: An emerging social problem. *Hospital and Community Psychiatry, 36,* 1063–1070.

Lewis, T. (2005). Altruism in classical Buddhism. In J. Neusner & B. Chilton (Eds.), *Altruism in world religions* (pp. 88–114). Washington, DC: Georgetown University Press.

Loukissa, D. A. (1995). Family burden in chronic mental illness: A review of research studies. *Journal of Advanced Nursing, 21,* 248–255.

Luks, A. (1988). Doing good: Helpers' high: Volunteering makes people feel good, physically and emotionally. *Psychology Today, 22(10),* 39, 42.

MacGregor, P. (1994). Grief: The unrecognized parental response to mental illness in a child. *Social Work, 39,* 160–166.

Maurin, J., & Boyd, C. (1990). Burden of mental illness on the family: A critical review. *Archives of Psychiatric Nursing, 4,* 99–107.

Meade, C. S. (2006). Sexual risk behavior among persons dually diagnosed with severe mental illness and substance use disorder. *Journal of Substance Abuse Treatment, 30,* 147–157.

Miller, F., Dworkin, J., Ward, M., & Barone, D. (1990). A preliminary study of unresolved grief in families of seriously mentally ill patients. *Hospital and Community Psychiatry, 41,* 1321–1325.

Miller, M. J., Denton, G. O., & Tobacyk, J. (1986). Social interest and feelings of hopelessness among elderly patients. *Psychological Reports, 58,* 410.

Musick, M., & Wilson, J. (2003). Volunteering and depression: The role of psychological and social resources in different age groups. *Social Science & Medicine, 56(2),* 259–269.

Neusner, J., & Avery-Peck, A. J. (2005). Altruism in classical Judaism. In J. Neusner & B. Chilton (Eds.), *Altruism in world religions* (pp. 31–52). Washington, DC: Georgetown University Press.

Neusner, J., & Chilton, B. (Eds.). (2005). *Altruism in world religions.* Washington, DC: Georgetown University Press.

Oman, D., Thoresen, C. E., & McMahon, K. (1999). Volunteerism and mortality among the community dwelling elderly. *Journal of Health Psychology, 4(3),* 301–316.

Post, S. (2008). Good to be good: Health and the generous heart. *Works of Love E-Newsletter,* Jan. 1, 1–24.

Potasznik, H., & Nelson, G. (1984). Stress and social support: The burden experienced by the family of a mentally ill person. *American Journal of Community Psychology, 12,* 589–607.

Reinhard, S. C., & Horwitz, A. V. (1995). Caregiver burden: Differentiating the content and consequences of family caregiving. *Journal of Marriage and the Family, 57,* 741–750.

Robinson, R. (Trans.). (1954). *Chinese Buddhist verse.* London: John Murray. Quoted in T. Lewis. (2005). Altruism in classical Buddhism. In J. Neusner & B. Chilton (Eds.), *Altruism in world religions* (pp. 88–114). Washington, DC: Georgetown University Press.

Schumann, H. W. (1973). *Buddhism: An outline of its teachings and schools.* (Trans. G. Feuerstein). Wheaton, IL: Quest Books.

Schwartz, C., Meisenhelder, J. B., Ma, Y., & Reed, G. (2003). Altruistic social interest behaviors are associated with better mental health. *Psychosomatic Medicine, 65,* 778–785.

Shih, H-C. (1994). *The sutra on Upasaka precepts.* Berkeley, CA: Numata Center for Buddhist Translation and Research. Quoted in T. Lewis. (2005). Altruism in classical Buddhism. In J. Neusner & B. Chilton (Eds.), *Altruism in world religions* (pp. 88–114). Washington, DC: Georgetown University Press.

Smith, H. (1991). *The world's religions: Our great wisdom traditions.* San Francisco: HarperSanFrancisco.

Steffen, P. R., & Masters, K. S. (2005). Does compassion mediate the religion-health relationship? *Annals of Behavioral Medicine, 30*(3), 217–224.

Thomson, E. H., Jr., & Doll, W. (1982). The burden of families coping with the mentally ill: An invisible crisis. *Family Relations, 31,* 379–388.

Unson, C., Mahoney-Trella, P., & Chowdhury, S. (2004). *Older African-American women's strategies for living long and healthy lives.* Paper presented at the Annual Meeting of the International Communication Association, New Orleans, Louisiana. Retrieved September 7, 2007, from http://www.allacademic.com/meta/p113094_index.html

Zarski, J. J., Bubenzer, D. L., & West, J. D. (1986). Social interest, stress, and the prediction of health status. *Journal of Consulting Development, 64,* 386–389.

SUGGESTIONS FOR FURTHER READING

Giving and Generosity

Post, S., & Newmark, J. (2007). *Why good things happen to good people.* New York: Broadway Books.

Salamon, J. (2003). *Rambam's ladder: A meditation on generosity and why it is necessary to give.* New York: Workman Publishing.

Helping Others as Self-Help

Kurtz, L. F. (1990). The self help movement: Review of the past decade of research. *Social Work with Groups: A Journal of Community and Clinical Practice, 13*(3), 101–115.

Kyrouz, E. H., Humphreys, K., & Loomis, C. (2002). A review of research on the effectiveness of self-help mutual aid groups. In B. J. White & E. J. Madara (Eds.), *The self-help group sourcebook: Your guide to community and online support* (7th ed., pp. 71–85). Denville, NJ: American Self-Help Clearinghouse, Department of St. Clares Health Services.

Mental Illness and the Family

Beard, J. J., & Gillespie, P. (2002). *Nothing to hide: Mental illness in the family.* New York: New Press.

Karp, D. A. (2001). *The burden of sympathy: How families cope with mental illness.* New York: Oxford University Press.

CHAPTER 9

The River:

Adapting to Change

RESILIENCY IN MENTAL HEALTH: A CRITICAL QUALITY

Research efforts are often focused on the identification of factors that may be associated with or predict individuals' vulnerability to adversity or illness. More recently, increased efforts are being made to understand resiliency: why and how some individuals, in comparison with others, are able to withstand and even flourish in the face of adverse circumstances (Buckley, Throngren, & Kleist, 1997; Watt, David, Ladd, & Shamos, 1995).

Numerous examples exist of the differences in individuals' abilities to address and overcome adverse circumstances and events. It appears, for instance, that females are less affected by parental alcoholism than are males (Latcham, 1985) and that females with schizophrenia tend to experience better outcomes over time than do their male counterparts (Seeman, 1986; Watt, Katz, & Shepard, 1983). Estimates from an epidemiological study indicate that approximately 90% of citizens in the United States are exposed to one or more traumatic events during their lifetimes (Yehuda, 1999), but only a fraction of those who are exposed to even the most severe traumatic events develop posttraumatic stress disorder (Yehuda, 1999; Yehuda, McFarlane, & Shalev, 1998). Women appear to be almost twice as likely as men to develop posttraumatic stress disorder following exposure to a traumatic event, regardless of the nature of the event (for example, rape, car crash, or physical assault) (Breslau, Chilcoat, Kessler, Peterson, & Lucia, 1999). And, although younger persons who have major depression have increased rates of suicidal ideation, the majority of depressed young people do not develop suicidal ideation or attempt suicide (Bostwick & Pankratz, 2000; Clark & Goebel-Fabbri, 1999; Kovacs, Goldston, & Gatsonis, 1993).

The quality of resiliency has been defined in a number of ways. Bonanno (2004, p. 20) has explained it as "the ability of adults in otherwise normal circumstances who are exposed to an isolated and potentially highly disruptive event . . . to maintain relatively stable, healthy levels of psychological and physical functioning." Redl (1969) hypothesized that resiliency comprises both an individual's capacity to withstand pathogenic pressures and his or her ability to recover from temporary collapse quickly and without assistance to return to a normal state of functioning. In other words, the extent to which an individual is resilient may be an important factor in how he or she processes and interprets traumatic events and what strategies he or she uses to assist in modifying adverse aspects of the environments and minimizing the internal sense of threat (Collins, Baum, & Singer, 1983; Ehlers, Maercker, & Boos, 2000; Green, Grace, & Gleser, 1985; Lindeman, Saari, Verkasalo, & Prytz, 1996).

The investigation into the specific nature and development of resiliency has occurred in three successive waves (Richardson, 2002). The first wave, which focused on the identification of resilient qualities, produced a listing of qualities and protective factors that were thought to help individuals overcome adversity. Individual-level factors that were found to be associated with greater resiliency include relatively higher levels of self-esteem (Fergusson, Beautrais, & Horwood, 2003), fortitude, determination, and self-assertion (Watt, David, et al., 1995); lower levels of novelty seeking (Fergusson & Lynskey, 1996); relatively higher levels of intelligence and greater problem solving skills (Herrenkohl, Herrenkohl, & Egolf, 1994; Kandel et al., 1988; Masten et al., 1988); a more easy-going temperament (Werner, 1989); and the ability to utilize environmental resources, such as counselors, to provide assistance in transcending adversity (Haldeman & Baker, 1992; Watt, David, et al., 1995). Family- and peer-level factors, such as a supportive relationship with at least one parent or parent-figure (Gribble et al., 1993; Seifer, Sameroff, Baldwin, & Baldwin, 1992) and good peer relationships (Werner, 1989), have also been found to be associated with resilience in children and adolescents. Werner (1989, p. 80) summarized what has come to be thought of as the characteristic triad of factors that contribute to resiliency in children and adults:

> Three types of protective factors emerge from our analyses of the developmental course of high-risk children from infancy to adulthood: 1) dispositional attributes of the individual, such as activity level and sociability, at least average intelligence, competence in communication skills (language and reading), and an internal locus of control; 2) affectional ties within the family that provide emotional support in times of stress, whether from a parent, sibling, spouse, or mate; and 3) external support systems, whether in school, at work, or church, that reward the individual's competencies and determination, and provide a belief system by which to live.

Rather than focusing on the identification of qualities, the second wave inquiry focused on an investigation into the process by which resilient qualities are acquired. Resiliency was no longer seen as the presence or absence of specified traits and characteristics, but instead as "the process of coping with stressors, adversity, change or opportunity in a manner that results in the identification, fortification, and enrichment of protective factors" (Richardson, 2002, p. 308). What this means is that individuals who have adapted physically, mentally, emotionally, and spiritually to their circumstances ("biopsychospiritual homeostasis") will nevertheless be confronted with various forms of change that may present as stressors, disruptions, events, or opportunities. Individuals will deal with these forms of change through one or more mechanisms of reintegration: by undergoing growth or developing new insights through an introspective process of identifying, accessing, and nurturing of resilient qualities ("resilient reintegration"); by attempting to return to their previous state of adaptation ("reintegration back to homeostasis"); by giving up hope or motivation ("recovering with loss"); or by resorting to self-destructive behaviors, such as substance use ("dysfunctional reintegration") (Richardson, 2002, pp. 311–312). This process occurs at the level of the individual, couple, family, and community. The time required to effectuate the process of reintegration varies across individuals and events. *What is critical is that individuals understand that they may choose how to respond to the potentially disruptive changes* (Richardson, 2002).

The third wave of the resilience inquiry has been termed resilience theory (Richardson, 2002). This theory rests on the assumption that "there is a force within everyone that drives them to self-actualization, altruism, wisdom, and harmony with a spiritual source of strength. This force is resilience . . ." (Richardson, 2002, p. 213). This phase of the inquiry focuses on discovering the client's internal source of strength and motivation.

The metaphor of the river can be used with clients in the context of each of these three aspects of resilience to assist them in their efforts to deal with change: to identify specific traits that contribute to their resilience; to identify, understand, and expand upon the strategies that they use to respond to life's changes; and to identify and expand their ability to draw upon their internal source of strength.

THE RIVER AND ITS MEANINGS

A Buddhist monk in Vietnam once said to me, "You never step into the same river twice." I considered this for some time. It is true that if you step into the river, step out, and then step in again, it is not the same river as it was even a second earlier, because the water that you previously stepped into has moved. But you are also not the same person as the individual who stepped into the river even a moment sooner; then, your foot was dry, and now it is wet. Even the shores that adjoin the river have changed. Perhaps they have slightly less soil because the river has washed some away, or perhaps there is slightly more as a result of deposits brought by the moving waters.

What I learned from this exchange is that change may be so imperceptible that we cannot measure it or even see it, but that does not mean that it has not occurred. When we approach a situation with which we are experiencing difficulty, we cannot assume that it is the same situation that we last faced, because time has passed and, with that passage of time, we have changed, other persons involved may have changed, and even the larger context may have changed.

Not surprisingly, the river has been utilized by writers as a symbol of change. For instance, in George Eliot's *The Mill on the Floss,* the Floss River appears as a force for change or a factor that promotes change (Makurath, 1975), a symbol of the "permanence of impermanence" (Knoepflmacher, cited in Makurath, 1975, p. 299). Hermann Hesse in *Siddhartha* utilized the river to signify internal change and growth, as illustrated in the following passages:

> It seemed to him that the river had something special to tell him, something he did not yet know, that still lay ahead of him. In this river Siddhartha had wanted to drown himself; in it today, the old, tired despairing Siddhartha had drowned. But the new Siddhartha felt a profound love toward this flowing stream and resolved not to leave it soon (Hesse, 2002, p. 105).

With change comes newness, however small the degree of newness may be. Many religions utilize water as a symbol of newness. In the Old Testament of the Bible, Genesis 6:6–9 tells the story of Noah, Noah's building of the ark, and the flood that God caused to ravage and destroy all creatures, with the exception of those whose safety had been secured on the ark. The eradication of almost all that had existed represented not only the ending of an epoch characterized by man's wickedness, but the beginning of a new era marked by a covenant between God and all life on earth.

In Christianity the act of baptism signifies not only a cleansing, but also the beginning of a life to be lived according to specified principles. By the third century, one's initiation into Christianity as an adult consisted of a one- to three-year period during which individuals learned the Christian way of life and how to refrain from engaging in self-destructive and socially harmful behaviors. This process ultimately culminated in a water bath and participation in the Eucharistic supper. The baptism in the water bath signified the individual's immersion into a new community and the initiation of a new life

(Haquin, 2006; Martos, 2005). Zoroastrianism also teaches of a Great Flood that destroyed the sinful world and the world's new beginning with the creatures that were saved by Yima following his construction of a *vara,* or sieve (Boyce, 2001). The themes of purification, life, and death, meaning new endings and new beginnings, appear frequently in rites and myths associated with the Ganges River, considered the holiest of India's rivers.

USING THE RIVER METAPHOR

Identifying Traits

Like the metaphor of the alphabet soup, the metaphor of the river can be used to identify specific traits that the client has utilized in the past. In contrast to the alphabet soup metaphor, though, I have used the river metaphor to help clients identify those specific traits that have helped them to deal with change in their lives. These may or may not be the same attributes that they select for their alphabet.

I have introduced the river metaphor as follows:

> Are you willing to try an experiment? If you are comfortable, close your eyes for just a few moments. Imagine that you are a river coursing through a river bed. Feel the speed that you are flowing and the texture of the river bed. Can you tell me what it is like being the river?

As the client shares with me his or her experience as a river, I may followup with various questions, depending on what the client has offered.

> How deep are you as a river? Can you see to the bottom?
> How fast are you moving? What does it feel like? Is it the right speed for you or do you want it to be different?
> Are you hitting any rough or scary spots? How do you handle that? What helps you get through those spots? Do you use these same strategies or qualities now? In what way?

Geoffrey, who you may remember from the chapter titled "The Alphabet Soup," had felt insecure and often unloved as a child because of the physical abuse that he had witnessed in his home and his rejection due to his homosexuality. His feelings of unworthiness were further exacerbated following the termination of his relationship with his partner of many years, his diagnosis of schizophrenia, and his subsequent loss of employment and bankruptcy. Like many individuals with schizophrenia, periods of dramatic change were quite difficult for Geoffrey.

I used the metaphor of the river with Geoffrey. Some clients may use the idea of the river as a reference point for their lives or for change itself. Still others may think of themselves as a river, coursing through the bed that was somehow created for them. Geoffrey immediately equated the river with his life and the constancy of change, remarking, "The only thing that is really permanent or sure is change itself."

Geoffrey enthusiastically listed those qualities that he believed helped him both survive and adapt to change and, sometimes, even flourish. He wrote:

The universe provides me with a new beginning every day.
Life is more than who I am.
Everything is temporary.
The universe provides enough change on a daily basis even when I don't feel motivated to bring about a change on my own, for example, the four seasons, the sun rising and setting, the change in trees.
The best I can hope for is to successfully manage my life, not control it.

When I asked Geoffrey if there were personality or character traits that gave rise to these perspectives, he thought about it for some time and then stated, "Unfounded optimism." This was, in fact, an accurate depiction of his approach to many situations. Geoffrey believed that, despite his daily struggles with varying levels of paranoia, the intermittent intrusion of voices in his head into his otherwise rational thought, and his ongoing financial worries, if he applied himself and worked hard to remain well, good things would follow. Upon further reflection, he was able to identify additional qualities that helped him deal successfully with change: flexibility, a sense of humor about himself and the larger world, and perseverance.

Identifying and Expanding Strategies

Wally, a semi-retired health professional in his mid-60s, faced a critical juncture in his relationship with his wife. They had been married for several decades and considered themselves to be blessed with each other, with their adult married children, and with the joy of their many grandchildren. Over the last few years, Wally's wife seemed to have developed some level of paranoia, believing that any unfindable misplaced item had been stolen, that her husband was being unfaithful, and that unnamed others were planning her demise. Stressors that she would have once characterized as minor annoyances became major traumas that sent her back to her bed for the remainder of the day. She became confused about the sequence of relatively recent events and the chronology of past and present. Ultimately, Crystal was diagnosed with early onset Alzheimer's disease.

Although the pronouncement of the diagnosis provided Wally with an explanation of the changes that he was seeing in his wife, it did little to provide him with a means of coping with these changes or their impact on their relationship. Where Crystal had once been supportive, she was now dependent, much as a young child might be. Where she was once generous in her praise of others and appreciative of their efforts and contributions, she was now critical and demanding. In the past, she had been affectionate and demonstrative; now, she engaged in angry tirades and frequently demanded reinforcement and praise from those in her family and social circle. Family members became increasingly uncertain how to respond to Crystal; her moods and behavior were inconsistent and unpredictable. Pleasurable moments with Wally and other family members became relatively infrequent, and the level of tension and conflict in their relationship grew.

Wally's confusion and the increasing level of conflict were not surprising in view of the ambiguity inherent in Crystal's condition and the situation as a whole. Wally was experiencing what has been called "ambiguous loss" (Boss, 1999), a term used to refer to situations in which a loved one continues to be psychologically present but is physically absent, such as when one's enlisted son is labeled "missing in action" during wartime, and situations in which the loved person continues to be physically present but is psychologically absent, as was the case with Crystal. Pauline Boss (1999, pp. 7–8) has explained why individuals may experience confusion and increased family conflict in such circumstances:

> First, because the loss is confusing, people are baffled and immobilized. They don't know how to make sense of the situation. They can't problem-solve because they do not yet know whether the problem (the loss) is final or temporary . . . Second, the uncertainty prevents people from adjusting to the ambiguity of their loss by reorganizing the roles and rules of their relationship with the loved one, so that the couple or family relationship freezes in place. If they have not already closed out the person who is missing physically or psychologically, they hang on to the hope that things will return to the way they used to be. Third, people are denied the symbolic rituals that ordinarily support a clear loss—such as a funeral after a death in the family . . . Fourth, the absurdity of ambiguous loss reminds people that life is not always rational or just; consequently, those who witness it tend to withdraw rather than give neighborly support . . . Finally, because ambiguous loss is a loss that goes on and on, those who experience it . . . become physically and emotionally exhausted from the relentless uncertainty.

Because ambiguous loss is continuous, individuals who experience such a loss are not able to detach or grieve and go on with their lives. Instead, they may feel stuck as if frozen in a time warp or in a freeze frame. What was once real may seem no longer real; their subjective experience of what had been their relationship can no longer be validated by their partner in that relationship.

Wally had a great deal of self-insight and an intellectual understanding of the probable trajectory of Crystal's illness. However, he had not incorporated either his awareness of his own strengths or his knowledge of Crystal's worsening condition into the strategies that he had tentatively formulated to help both himself and Crystal through her process of deterioration. We talked about change and the nature of change, relating this to the metaphor of the river. Just as change in the color, volume, or texture of the water may be imperceptible, so too may changes in mental status and in relationships be almost imperceptible and immeasurable. Just as the intensity of the water's movement may change unpredictably, now meandering calmly only to later surge violently, so too can an illness progress slowly or rapidly, and the rapidity of that course cannot be predicted.

Wally knew what he believed his greatest strengths to be: creativity, a sense of humor, a need for human contact and affiliation, a sense of responsibility, long-term friendships. He had used various strategies in the past to cope with periods of adversity: reliance on his sense of humor to make things seem not so bad, creative problem-solving to design solutions to troubling situations, reaching out to friends for support. How, then, could these strategies be expanded in order to cope better with the changes in Crystal's behavior and in their relationship?

Wally was able to identify several ways in which he could capitalize on his strengths and extend his previously used strategies to formulate additional and expanded coping strategies. His part-time work at a local social service organization provided him with professional companionship, intellectual stimulation, and a sense of vitality. Although he had considered increasing the number of hours that he spent there each week, he was concerned that doing so would prevent him from enjoying the amount of time available to him to enjoy Crystal's company in her more lucid moments. Additionally, although his work with clients challenged him intellectually, it was frequently emotionally draining, and Wally did not feel that he had any extra energy. Wally had always wanted to write; in fact, he had once fantasized about becoming a journalist or novelist. This might be the perfect opportunity to begin his venture into creative writing. The creative endeavor would be intellectually stimulating and, if he worked at home on his computer, he would be able to spend more time with Crystal. Conference calls from home could provide him with additional professional interaction.

Although Wally would have liked to have someone come in to the house each week to help with the cleaning, he did not believe that this arrangement would be wise in view of Crystal's level of paranoia. Instead, he enlisted the assistance of several nearby friends and relatives. This provided him with a reprieve from the expenditure of yet more energy for housework, and also provided both him and Crystal with additional companionship.

Finding Internal Strength

Individuals who are feeling anxious, depressed, troubled, or worried from the onslaught of events in their daily lives may wonder whether they have the strength to make it through the difficult times. They may experience moments of hopelessness, some brief, some seemingly never-ending. Rapid and sudden change in life circumstances may provoke such feelings or exacerbate already-existing feelings of despair. Yet, most people do make it through, much as water continues to flow, sometimes mightily, sometimes as a mere trickle, despite storms, droughts, even human interference. How do they do this?

Many people draw on their religious or spiritual beliefs and practices as a source of strength. Although concepts of religiosity and spirituality have often been used interchangeably (O'Neill & Kenny, 1998), distinctions have been made between the two. Spirituality is often thought of as a focus on God or other power that guides the universe, faith in mystical or transcendental experiences, and/or adherence to certain moral values and belief about relationships with people and a higher power (Mathew, Georgi, Wilson, & Mathew, 1996; Warfield & Goldstein, 1996). Spirituality has been conceived of as "a basic aspect of human existence . . . [that] encompasses human activities of moral decision making, searching for a sense of meaning and purpose in life, and striving for mutually fulfilling relationships among individuals, society and ultimate reality, however conceptualized" (Canda, 1988, p. 238); "one's personalized experience . . . pertaining to a sense of worth, meaning, vitality, and connectedness to others and the universe" (Titone, 1991, p. 8); and "a striving for and infusion with the reality of the interconnectedness among self, other people, and the Infinite/Divine" (Ingersoll, 1994, p. 102). In contrast, religion has been said to represent "the external expression of faith (the inner beliefs and values that relate the person to the transcendent or God). It is comprised [sic] of beliefs, ethical codes, and worship practices that unite an individual with a moral community" (Joseph, 1988, p. 444). Spirituality and religion have also been viewed as two dimensions of the same construct, with spirituality representing the inward, individual experience and religion signifying the external manifestation of that experience (Fowler, 1981).

Not surprisingly, individuals with diagnoses of a severe mental illness may also find that their sense of inner strength derives from their spiritual and religious beliefs. Religious and spiritual activities, such as prayer, attendance at religious services, meditation, study of the scriptures, and meetings with a spiritual leader, have been found to have positive effects on individuals' management of their mental illness symptoms (Loue & Sajatovic, 2006; Mitchell & Romans, 2003; Tepper, Rogers, Coleman, & Malony, 2001). For instance, one woman who participated in a study that examined HIV risk among women with schizophrenia, bipolar disorder, and major depression explained how she relied on God to help her feel better:

> God tells you not to worry about tomorrow because tomorrow is not promised. The birds don't have any clothes but God provides. We are his children and he will provide. Sometimes we feel sad because we are human, but you ask God and you will feel better (Loue & Sajatovic, 2006, p. 1175).

As indicated above, Geoffrey and I had worked together over time to identify Geoffrey's strengths and how he had used them and could continue to use them to address any variety of situations that he might face. It was also important, however, that Geoffrey be able to identify an internal source of strength upon which he could draw for renewal and support. Geoffrey had relatively few external supports upon which he could rely, which made this even more critical.

We used the metaphor of the winding, changing river to identify periods in Geoffrey's life when he felt particularly strong. Geoffrey remembered back to when he was a child finding himself at the end of a rainbow that was formed following a storm. He interpreted the sign of the rainbow and its presence near him as a sign from God that, despite whatever others might say about him, he was God's child and was loved and would endure despite any adverse events that might arise in his life. With his permission, Geoffrey's poem about this experience and the inner strength that he derives from it is reprinted here:

Rainbow's End: A Testimonial
Once, I stood at the end of a rainbow
certain God made me the pot of gold
Believing all that I felt
was what mattered
Never minding that which
I was told.
Being chosen has not made
me better than others
But with so many auras
How could one go wrong?
By painting life with the shades of that long-ago rainbow
Has ensured me a place in the sun.

REFERENCES

Bonanno, G. A. (2004). Loss, trauma, and human resilience: Have we underestimated the human capacity to thrive after extremely aversive events? *American Psychologist, 59*(1), 20–28.

Boss, P. (1999). *Ambiguous loss: Learning to live with unresolved grief.* Cambridge, MA: Harvard University Press.

Bostwick, J. M., & Pankratz, V. S. (2000). Affective disorders and suicide risk: A reexamination. *American Journal of Psychiatry, 157,* 1925–1932.

Boyce, M. (2001). *Zoroastrians: Their religious beliefs and practices.* London: Routledge.

Breslau, N., Chilcoat, H. D., Kessler, R. C., Peterson, E. L., & Lucia, V. C. (1999). Vulnerability to assaultive violence: Further specification of the sex difference in post-traumatic stress disorder. *Psychological Medicine, 29,* 813–821.

Buckley, M. R., Thorngren, J. M., & Kleist, D. M. (1997). Family resiliency: A neglected family construct. *The Family Journal: Counseling and Therapy for Couples and Families, 5*(3), 241–246.

Canda, E. R. (1988). Spirituality, religious diversity, and social work practice. *Social Casework: The Journal of Contemporary Social Work, 69*(4), 238–247.

Clark, D. C. & Goebel-Fabbri, A. E. (1999). Lifetime risk of suicide in major affective disorders. In D. G. Jacobs (Ed.), *Guide to suicide assessment and intervention* (pp. 270–286). San Francisco: Jossey-Bass Publishers.

Collins, D. L., Baum, A., & Singer, J. E. (1983). Coping with chronic stress at Three Mile Island: Psychological and biochemical evidence. *Psychology, 2,* 149–166.

Ehlers, A., Maercker, A., & Boos, A. (2000). Posttraumatic stress disorder following political imprisonment: The role of mental defeat, alienation, and perceived permanent change. *Journal of Abnormal Psychology, 109,* 45–55.

Eliot, George. (2002). *The mill on the Floss.* New York: Penguin.

Fergusson, D. M., Beautrais, A. L., & Horwood, L. J. (2003). Vulnerability and resiliency to suicidal behaviours in young people. *Psychological Medicine, 33,* 61–73.

Fergusson, D. M., & Lynskey, M. T. (1996). Adolescent resiliency to family adversity. *Journal of Child Psychology and Psychiatry, 37*(3), 281–292.

Fowler, J. W. (1981). *Stages of faith: The psychology of human development and the quest for meaning.* San Francisco: Harper and Row.

Green, B. L., Grace, M. C., & Gleser, G. (1985). Identifying survivors at risk: Long-term impairment following the Beverly Hills Supper Club fire. *Journal of Consulting and Clinical Psychology, 53,* 672–678.

Gribble, P. A., Cowen, E. L., Wyman, P. A., Work, W. C., Wannon, M., & Raoof, A. (1993). Parent and child views of parent-child relationship qualities and resilient outcomes among urban children. *Journal of Child Psychology and Psychiatry, 34,* 507–520.

Haldeman, D. E., & Baker, S. B. (1992). Helping female adolescents prepare to cope with irrational thinking via preventive cognitive self-instruction training. *Journal of Primary Prevention, 13,* 161–169.

Haquin, A. (2006). The liturgical movement and Catholic ritual revision. In G. Wainwright & K. B. Westerfield Tucker (Eds.). *The Oxford history of Christian worship* (pp. 696–720). New York: Oxford University Press.

Herrenkohl, E. C., Herrenkohl, R. C., & Egolf, B. (1994). Resilient early school-age children from maltreating homes: Outcomes in late adolescence. *American Journal of Orthopsychiatry, 64,* 301–309.

Hesse, H. (2002). *Siddhartha.* (trans. S.C. Cohn). Boston: Shambala.

Ingersoll, R. E. (1994). Spirituality, religion, and counseling: Dimensions and relationships. *Counseling and Values, 38(2),* 98–111.

Joseph, M. V. (1988). Religion and social work practice. *Social Casework: The Journal of Contemporary Social Work, 69(7),* 443–452.

Kandel, E., Mednick, S. A., Kirkegaard-Sorenson, L., Hutchings, B., Knop, J., Rosenberg, R., et al. (1988). IQ as a protective factor for subjects at high risk for antisocial behaviour. *Journal of Consulting and Clinical Psychology, 56,* 224–226.

Kovacs, M., Goldston, D., & Gatsonis, C. (1993). Suicidal behaviors and childhood-onset depressive disorders: A longitudinal investigations. *Journal of the American Academy of Child and Adolescent Psychiatry, 32,* 8–20.

Latcham, R. W. (1981). Familial alcoholism: Evidence from 237 alcoholics. *British Journal of Psychiatry, 147,* 54–57.

Lindeman, M., Saari, S., Verkasalo, M., & Prytz, H. (1996). Traumatic stress and its risk factors among peripheral victims of the M/S *Estonia* disaster. *European Psychology, 1,* 255–270.

Loue, S., & Sajatovic, M. (2006). Spirituality, coping, and HIV risk and prevention in a sample of severely mentally ill Puerto Rican women. *Journal of Urban Health, 83(6),* 1168–1182.

Makaruth, P. A., Jr. (1975). The symbolism of the flood in Eliot's *Mill on the Floss. Studies in the Novel, 7(2),* 298–300.

Martos, J. (2005). Sacraments. In J. Bowden (Ed.), *Encyclopedia of Christianity* (pp. 1060–1071). New York: Oxford University Press.

Masten, A. S., Garmezy, N., Tellegen, A., Pellegrini, D. S., Larkin, K., & Larsen, A. (1988). Competence and stress in school children: The moderating effects of individual and family qualities. *Journal of Child Psychology and Psychiatry, 29,* 745–764.

Mathew, R. J., Georgi, J., Wilson, W. H., & Mathew, V. G. (1996). A retrospective study of the concept of spirituality as understood by recovering individuals. *Journal of Substance Abuse Treatment, 13,* 67–73.

Mitchell, L., & Romans, S. (2003). Spiritual beliefs in bipolar affective disorder: Their relevance for illness management. *Journal of Affective Disorders, 75,* 247–257.

O'Neill, D. P., & Kenny, E. K. (1998). Spirituality and chronic illness. *Image: Journal of Nursing Scholarship, 30*(3), 275–280.

Redl, F. (1969). Adolescents—just how do they react? In G. Caplan & S. Lebovci (Eds.), *Adolescence: Psychosocial perspectives.* New York: Basic Books.

Richardson, G. E. (2002). The metatheory of resilience and resiliency. *Journal of Clinical Psychology, 58*(3), 307–321.

Seeman, M. V. (1986). Current outcome in schizophrenia: women versus men. *Acta Psychiatrica Scandinavica, 73,* 609–617.

Seifer, R., Sameroff, A. J., Baldwin, C. P., & Baldwin, A. (1992). Child and family factors that ameliorate risk between 4 and 13 years of age. *Journal of the American Academy of Child and Adolescent Psychiatry, 31,* 893–903.

Tepper, L., Rogers, S. A., Coleman, E. M., & Malony, H. N. (2001). The prevalence of religious coping among persons with persistent mental illness. *Psychiatric Services, 52*(5), 660–665.

Titone, A. (1991). Spirituality and psychotherapy in social work practice. *Spirituality and Social Work Communicator, 2*(1), 7–9.

Warfield, R. D., & Goldstein, M. B. (1996). Spirituality: The key to recovery from alcoholism. *Counseling and Values, 40,* 196–205.

Watt, N. F., David, J. P., Ladd, K. L., & Shamos, S. (1995). The life course of psychological resilience: A phenomenological perspective on deflecting life's slings and arrows. *Journal of Primary Prevention, 15,* 209–246.

Watt, D. C., Katz, K., & Shepard, M. (1983). The natural history of schizophrenia: A five year prospective follow-up of a representative sample of schizophrenics by means of a standardized clinical and social assessment. *Psychological Medicine, 13,* 663–670.

Werner, E. (1989). High risk children in young adulthood: A longitudinal study from birth to 32 years. *American Journal of Orthopsychiatry, 59,* 72–81.

Yehuda, R. (1999). Biological factors associated with susceptibility to posttraumatic stress disorder. *Canadian Journal of Psychiatry, 44,* 34–39.

Yehuda, R., McFarlane, A. C., & Shalev, A. Y. (1998). Predicting the development of posttraumatic stress disorder from the acute response to a traumatic event. *Biological Psychiatry, 44,* 1305–1313.

SUGGESTIONS FOR FURTHER READING

Illness and Loss

Gilbert, S. M. (2006). *Death's door: Modern dying and the way we grieve.* New York: W. W. Norton & Company.

Post, S. G. (2002). *The moral challenge of Alzheimer disease* (2nd ed.). Baltimore: Johns Hopkins University Press.

Religion, Spirituality, and Health

Koening, H. G., McCullough, M. E., & Larson, D. B. (2001). *Handbook of religion and health.* New York: Oxford University Press.

Koening, H. G. (Ed.). (1998). *Handbook of religion and mental health.* San Diego, CA: Academic Press.

Trauma

Levine, P. A. (1997). *Waking the tiger: Healing trauma.* Berkeley, CA: North Atlantic Books.

Vasterling, J. J., & Brewin, C. R. (Eds.). (2005). *Neuropsychology of PTSD: Biological, cognitive, and clinical perspectives.* New York: Guilford Press.

CHAPTER 10

The Tree:

Finding Self, Understanding Relationships

THE TREE: "THE SWISS ARMY KNIFE OF METAPHORS"

Each of the previous chapters focused on the use of a specific metaphor for a specific purpose or in a specific context. However, the use of a metaphor need not be constrained; the use of a specific metaphor is restricted only by the limits of one's own creativity. This chapter demonstrates how a specific metaphor, that of the tree, can be used for a variety of purposes, analogous to the use of a Swiss army knife for a multitude of tasks.

THE STORY OF THE TREE

The tree has stood for many things throughout cultures and traditions. Some of the meanings that are most familiar to Western readers come to us from the Bible. In Genesis 2:9, the Bible states,

> And out of the ground the Lord God made to grow every tree that is pleasant to the sight and good for food, the tree of life also in the midst of the garden, and the tree of knowledge of good and evil.

We see from this that the tree can symbolize sustenance of the spirit and the body ("pleasant to the sight and good for food"); development, growth, and mortality ("the tree of life"); and sustenance of the body, heart, and soul through the attainment of knowledge and wisdom ("tree of knowledge of good and evil").

Other portions of the Bible reinforce the significance of the tree as a source of nourishment. For instance, Deuteronomy 8:7–8 tells us of the Promised Land, that it is

> A good land with flowing streams, with springs and underground waters welling up in valleys and hills, a land of wheat and barley, of vines and *fig trees* and pomegranates, a land of *olive trees* and honey, a land where you may eat bread without scarcity (Smith, 1991, p. 278) (emphasis added).

Yogic tradition similarly analogizes the growth of the tree to the development of the self. Iyengar (2002, p. 7) tells us:

> When you grow a plant you first dig the earth, remove the stones and weeds and make the ground soft. Then you put the seed into the ground and surround it with the soft earth so carefully that when the seed opens it will not be damaged by the weight of the earth. Finally, you water the seed a little and wait for it to germinate and grow. After one or two days, the seed opens into a seedling and a stem grows from it. Then the stem splits into two branches and produces leaves. It steadily grows into a trunk and produces branches in various directions with many leaves.

> Similarly, the tree of the self needs to be taken care of. . . .

The development of the self is further analogized to the various parts of the tree. The roots represent freedom from various tendencies; the trunk signifies the strength that comes from adherence to various principles and practices; the branches stand for the postures that are utilized to bring into harmony the body's physical and physiological functions with yogic psychology. The leaves, bark, sap, and flower of the tree similarly represent different various aspects of our individual growth. Finally, the fruit of the tree signifies the culmination of the individual's growth: the unity of the body, mind, and soul merging with the Universal Spirit (Iyengar, 2002). Antoine de Saint-Exupéry's description of the growth of the tree evokes a similar image of the individual seeking to attain enlightenment: "The tree is more than first a seed, then a stem, then a living trunk, and then dead timber. The tree is a slow enduring force, straining to win the sky" (*The Wisdom of the Sands,* quoted in de Saint-Exupéry, 2002, p. 53).

Buddhism, too, utilizes the tree as a symbol for individual growth. It was under the Bodhi tree that the Buddha achieved enlightenment (Schumann, 1973; Smith, 1991). The Buddha, born as Siddhartha, was raised in a sheltered environment characterized by pleasure, luxury, and comfort, a world far removed from the pain, suffering, and death that people experienced in their lives (Snelling, 1991). On four successive occasions following his marriage and the birth of his son, Siddhartha wandered forth from his sheltered life into the larger world. It was on each of these journeys that he witnessed other aspects of life: an old man, a sick man, a corpse, and a holy man.

Siddhartha, now disenchanted with his life of ease and luxury and newly cognizant of the suffering inherent in human existence, left his home and his family. He renounced everything and assumed a life of asceticism, which ultimately provided no greater resolution to the problem of human suffering than had his previous life of luxury. Siddhartha seated himself beneath the bodhi tree, to remain there until he had discovered an answer to the problem of suffering. It was under this tree that Siddhartha was able to discard his attachment to his "I" and identify with his true nature. Siddhartha rose from his meditation as The Buddha: The Awakened One (Snelling, 1991).

Judaism has also used the image of the tree to signify wisdom, stating in the Talmud, "Wisdom is a tree and active virtue is its fruit" (Lankevich, 2002, p. 134). Yet another portion of the Talmud relies on the image of the tree to help us to understand how we establish our interconnectedness with others through deed:

> When our learning exceeds our deeds we are like trees whose branches are many but whose roots are few: the wind comes and uproots them. . . . But when our deeds exceed our learning we are like trees whose branches are few but whose roots are many, so that even if all the winds of the world were to come and blow against them, they would be unable to move them (Novak, 1994, p. 215).

It is our deeds, our actions toward and with others, that keep us rooted and connected and fulfill our need for affiliation.

The symbolism underlying Christianity's Jesse Tree reflects both connection and the attainment of knowledge and wisdom. It depicts Jesus' lineage that begins with Jesse, the father of David, and extends through the ancestors of Christ, depicted as its fruit. In essence, it is a family tree of Christ (Catholic Culture, 2008). The symbol of the Jesse Tree is premised on Isaiah 11:1–3:

> A shoot will come up from the stump of Jesse;
> From his roots a Branch will bear fruit.
> The Spirit of the Lord will rest on him—
> The Spirit of wisdom and understanding,
> The Spirit of counsel and of power,
> The Spirit of knowledge and of the fear of the Lord—
> And he will delight in the fear of the Lord.

The various symbols that adorn the Jesse Tree include the sun, signifying the light and eternal life that Jesus brings to dispel darkness; Jacob's ladder, symbolizing the ladder between heaven and earth (see Chapter 6 for additional discussion of Jacob's ladder); and the burning bush, used as a symbol here of the Virgin Birth of Christ because God appeared to Moses in the desert as a bush that burned but was not consumed (Catholic Culture, 2008). Because of the great significance of the Jesse Tree, it has been widely depicted in Christian art and examples can be found in many churches, including Dorchester Abbey in Oxfordshire, UK; Saint-Étienne Church in Beauvais, France; Cathedral Notre-Dame in Clement-Ferrand, France; the Church of Saint Francis in Oporto, Portugal; and Saint Louis Abbey in St. Louis, Missouri.

Other traditions bring us other meanings. It has been suggested that different types of trees signified specific periods or seasons of time in Celtic cosmology, with each type of tree referring to a specific god and having a specific meaning. As an example, the willow tree was said to correspond to the Celtic period known as Saille and is considered to be a tree of enchantment (Elgood, 1999). The acacia tree has been venerated across various cultures and eras as a symbol of the vernal equinox; a representation of purity and innocence because it shrinks from touch; and as the typification of human immortality, regeneration, and man's survival after the destruction of his visible nature (Hall, 2003).

Trees were widely worshipped across ancient cultures as proxies for the Divine; oaks, elms, and cedars, in particular, became symbols of divine protection, power, integrity, permanence, and virility (Hall, 2003). Trees and their associated male and female spirits have been worshipped in rural India (Elgood, 1999). The practice of preaching under a tree is an ancient one in India; the custom provides shade to the teachers and is said to facilitate the teacher's connection to the spirit of the sacred tree (Elgood, 1999). Planting peace trees is a common practice throughout various Asian cultures and traditions; the planting of a tree is believed to bring peace and reduce violence in the regions neighboring the tree.

USING THE METAPHOR

Using the Tree to Enhance Self-Understanding and Self-Development: The Tree of Knowledge and Enlightenment

I have suggested to clients with whom I have worked, both on an individual basis and in group, to visualize what they would look like as a tree. Not infrequently, individuals can picture in their minds what they might look like, or the tree that they might be, without knowing the name of the specific type of tree. Their image of the tree is a symbol for themselves and can then be used as a vehicle to explore their own qualities. And, because trees grow, the image of the tree can also be used with the client to explore the various dimensions of their current growth—physical, emotional, spiritual, and intellectual—and how they might like to grow in the future.

This visualization exercise can also be used together with techniques derived from person-centered expressive arts therapy. This approach involves the use of movement, drawing, painting, music, writing, and other forms of creative activity "in a supportive, client-centered setting" that allows the client to experience and express his or her feelings; this creative process is critical to the healing process (Rogers, 2001, p. 163). Expressive arts therapy rests on the assumption that every individual has worth, dignity, the capacity for self-direction, and a natural impulse towards growth. Empathic understanding is key:

> Empathic understanding means that the therapist senses accurately the feelings and personal meanings that the client is experiencing and communicates this acceptant understanding to the client. When functioning best, the therapist is so much inside the private world of the other that he/she can clarify not only the meanings of which the client is aware but even those just below the level of awareness. Listening of this very special, active kind, is one of the most potent forces for change . . . (Kirschenbaum & Henderson, 1989, p. 136).

I introduce the use of the tree metaphor in group by explaining that throughout history, individuals and cultures have identified with trees. I then ask the clients why they think that might be. I try to avoid giving as much detail about the symbolism of the tree as I have here until the end of the group, in order to avoid the possibility that I might steer clients' thinking in a particular direction. Following this very brief introduction and some discussion by the clients, I make available an assortment of materials that the clients can use to produce their trees.

Clients can use any of various materials—paper, paint, crayons, pens, pencils—to illustrate the tree that they would be. The client then uses the drawing as a point of reference. For instance, they may describe the various parts of the tree and how these parts relate to the client him- or herself, or by telling a story about the tree, that they then use as a vehicle to discuss their own story.

One man, whom I will call Frank, began his story of himself as a tree by stating flatly that he could not draw. Nevertheless, he attempted to draw a portrait of Frank as a Tree. His crayoned picture showed a small, skinny little thing off in the bottom right-hand corner of the large piece of paper that he had selected. "I just can't draw," he said, seemingly defeatedly, but also with a note of protest and accusation in his voice.

"What do you see there?" I asked. "Does your tree have a message for you?"

As Frank told his story, it became increasingly clear how he resembled the tree that he had drawn. Frank, in his 70s, had been suffering from major depression for an extended period of time. Despite his divorce from his wife of many years, she continued to care about him deeply and attended both individual and group therapy sessions with him in an effort to support him in his treatment. Frank lived with one of his adult daughters who, he was convinced, felt burdened by his presence, although she had never indicated this by either word or deed. Frank claimed that he could feel only a heavy tiredness that seemed both impenetrable and never-ending. He had no strengths, he said; his tree was visibly shrunken and wilted.

The group pointed out to Frank that he did, indeed, have strength. Despite his despondency, his lack of vibrancy, and the depth of his despair, he managed to find the energy and strength within himself to attend group every morning. He helped his daughter with her household chores, such as washing dishes. He was sufficiently aware of himself and others to be able to identify who in his network of friends and family members would be willing and able to support him through his treatment for depression and to ask them for and rely on them for assistance.

I asked Frank how he would describe his tree after having received this feedback from other group members. Would it be the same or had it changed? It had, indeed, changed, according to Frank's description. Although still ungrounded with no root system, Frank described it as taller and rounder, with maybe a few leaves. If only momentarily, Frank had begun to feel his strength. It would be critical in the future for him to continue to identify, feel, and utilize this and other strengths and abilities.

Using the Tree to Understand Our Interconnectedness and Relationships: The Tree of Nourishment

The tree can also be used as a metaphor for one's relationships with others. This is how Marshall, a middle-aged man, utilized his image of the tree. Marshall had recently been diagnosed with bipolar disorder and was in the process of sorting through numerous legal problems that stemmed from his violent behaviors. Although Marshall's episodic violence towards his family members may have been associated in part with his bipolar disorder, he was unable to see that what he had done was, in fact, violence and that he, not his family members, was responsible for the behavior that had led to these legal difficulties.

Marshall saw himself as a leaf on the tree. He was situated very close to other leaves on the tree, in fact, "too close." He did not want to be so close to these other leaves, but instead wanted "space" and "freedom." "When the other leaves get too close, I get angry," he said. And, even though Marshall the Leaf wanted "space" from the other leaves, he wanted "to control them." "They do what they want, they fall off, they go away, they don't listen to me." Even though Marshall wanted his "space" and his "freedom," the space was to be created on his terms; when the other leaves left of their own accord, it was an event out of his control and he became angry.

I asked Marshall what it was that connected him to these other leaves, since they were on the same tree and some were even on the same branch and, hence, their closeness. "I give them guidance, they can learn from me." "Do you feel anything toward them or they toward you?" I asked. "I want them to leave me alone," Marshall said. "It's too much responsibility."

Here, then, was a clue to what Marshall had been feeling and had been unable to voice directly. Perhaps he had felt for some time that he had had to shoulder too much of the responsibility for his family's well-being, or perhaps the increasingly present mental illness had lowered his threshold for tolerating stress, a not uncommon corollary of severe mental illness (Bybee, Mowbray, Oyserman, & Lewandowski, 2006; Torrey & Knable, 2002).

Whatever the reason, it was clear that this was an issue that would require attention not only from Marshall but from other family members as well. Marshall's use of the tree as a metaphor for his relationships provided an opening for this discussion with his wife and teen-age children. Unlike older models of treatment for mental illness that had operated from the perspective of the "patient being treated for a chronic illness" (Glynn, Cohen, Dixon, & Niv, 2006), the outpatient program that Marshall was attending welcomed the participation of family members as part of the treatment process, with the attendee's consent.

The participation of Marshall's family members in the treatment process was potentially critical to Marshall's recovery from this acute episode of illness in a number of ways. First, there were clearly issues involving the entire family. Resolution would require clear communication (Satir, 1964, 1972) and potentially a realignment of roles within the family unit, such as the allocation of responsibilities. A unilateral decision by Marshall to ignore stressful, but important, responsibilities would likely impact other members of his family system (Bertalanffy, 1968).

Second, individuals with bipolar disorder frequently do not adhere to their prescribed medication regimens (Lingam & Scott, 2002; Perlick, Rosenheck, Kaczynski, & Kozma, 2004). In fact, one of the most difficult and pervasive obstacles to good outcomes among individuals with serious mental illness, including individuals with bipolar disorder, is their premature discontinuation of medications (Begley et al., 2001; Colom, Vieta, Tacci, Sanchez-Moreno, & Scott, 2005; Lieberman et al., 2005; Lingam & Scott, 2002; Osterberg & Blaschke, 2005). Individuals who are supported and accepted by family members may be more likely to utilize mental health services appropriately (Pescosolido, Gardner, & Lubell, 1998) and may be less likely to experience a relapse (Miklowitz & Goldstein, 1990). Positive family interactions and good support may also have a favorable effect on illness behavior including better coping with illness, modulation of guilt/shame, and development of a hopeful perspective, increased sense of competence, and better self-esteem (Johnson, Meyer, Winnett, & Small, 2000).

Some might argue against the participation of Marshall's family members in the treatment process specifically because of Marshall's past enraged outbursts and threats of bodily harm directed against his wife and daughters (Austin & Dankwort, 1999). This may stem from a belief that the acceptance of personal responsibility for one's violence or threatened violence is paramount (Dutton & Golant, 1995) and that the inclusion of family members in therapy with the individual too easily allows him or her to avoid personal responsibility and use the actions of the family members as an excuse for his or her violent threats and actions. Some clinicians may fear that the participation of threatened or harmed family members in the treatment of their threatening family member may lead them to believe erroneously that they are responsible for the individual's inability to respond nonthreateningly and nonviolently (Felder & Victor, 1996). In Marshall's situation, for example, the concern might be that the inclusion of family members in the treatment process would allow Marshall to rationalize his violent threats as a justifiable response to what he perceived as his family's excessive demands on his time and energy, or that his family members would come to believe that they were responsible for Marshall's threats.

Other clinicians and researchers have objected to the inclusion of the threatened family member(s) in the treatment process with the threatening individual because the openness required of the threatened individual might actually increase their risk of harm (Gondolf & Russell, 1986). In a situation such as Marshall's, the risk of potential harm to his family members that could occur as the result of their involvement in the treatment process must be balanced against the potential benefits both to the family members and to Marshall.

Karen's use of the tree metaphor provides another illustration of how the tree metaphor can be used both to identify clients' strengths and the nature of their relationships with others. Karen was a participant in a group for individuals who had been suffering from depression. She had found it increasingly difficult to work because of her symptoms and had ultimately taken a leave of absence from work to participate in an intensive outpatient therapy program. Karen used the metaphor of the tree to describe both herself and her relationships to those around her:

> I am beautiful. I am caring, see, I give shade to people. I am also supportive. I am open, my branches spread wide. I am giving. The birds come and rest on my branches. There is newness in me, with these leaves.

When asked what the birds meant to her, Karen spoke of her children and husband and how she provided them with support and how they helped make her happy. The ability to give to others, Karen believed, was one of her greatest strengths and grew directly from her belief in God and God's goodness.

Karen's identification of the mutual support that she and her family members give to each other provided her with knowledge that she would be able to use in the future if she were to find herself becoming depressed. Research has demonstrated that a support network and connection with others may be critical to maintaining good mental health and avoiding relapse (Bloch & Singh, 1997; Torrey & Knable, 2002).

The metaphor of the tree can also be used as a template for the construction of a family or community genogram. Genograms are often used to help clients develop an understanding of how they evolve in relation to others, their connectedness to others, and the degree of power and influence exerted by various individuals, groups, and entities that constitute their world (Ivey, 1998; Rigazio-DiGilio, Ivey, Kunkler-Peck, & Grady, 2005). The client's definition of his or her network as a tree also provides the counselor or therapist with important information about the strengths that the client may be able to draw upon from diverse sources.

The use of the genogram tree with Sara illustrates how this can be used with a client. Sara, a middle-class woman in her 30s, had been previously diagnosed with an adjustment disorder. She had been raised by parents who were both rigid and intermittently volatile, sometimes resulting in physical and emotional abuse directed at Sara and her siblings. Sara's parents responded to her sexual abuse by a friend of the family when she was 11 by blaming her. They continued to have the family friend drive Sara to her after-school activities despite her protestations. Sara's parents responded to her attempts to run away in an effort to avoid further abuse with angry outcries about her lack of consideration.

Sara came to counseling feeling not just that she was disconnected from others but that she had no connection with anyone or anything. We gradually began to examine her connections by using the metaphor of the tree and ultimately using the tree to display her genogram. Her roots became her strong connection to her faith and the traditions of her grandparents, who had migrated to the United States from Europe. Her branches became her arms that reached out and connected her to the world around her—other trees, birds, the sky, the sun, each of which represented a significant figure or entity in her life. The leaves both protected her trunk—her inner core—and became her manner of presentation to the world. Sara recognized that she could change her presentation, much as a tree's appearance reflects the change of seasons through the transformation, death, and re-emergence of its leaves. Some branches were stronger than others, and some leaves more glorious than others. Ultimately, the construction of the tree-as-genogram enabled Sara to recognize and acknowledge Sara-in-context.

Using the Tree to Visualize the Future: The Tree of Enchantment

As was discussed in great detail in Chapter 4, individuals have the potential to achieve self-actualization, that is, "the full use and exploitation of [their] talents, capacities, potentialities" once their more basic biological and affiliations needs have been met (Maslow, 1970, p. 150). The process of attaining self-actualization has been likened to the growth of a tree:

> What is needed for self-actualization to proceed successfully is a nurturing environment that provides adequate sustenance and social support, as well as a personal commitment to growth. Self-actualization is like the process of an oak growing from a seed into a full tree. The acorn seed already has within it the potential for the full oak, but adequate sunlight, water, nutrient and other environmental supports are necessary for the growth to occur. On the one hand, development is like the natural emergence and expansive growth upward of the inborn potentials (self-actualization). On the other hand, development is like the tree striving up toward the light, as when people seek fulfillment by stretching toward their own ideals and aspirations and toward loving and responsible connections with others (Robbins, Chatterjee, & Canda, 1998, p. 362).

I have found that clients are particularly receptive to the idea of a tree of enchantment near the holidays in December, perhaps because of our culture's focus on the Christmas tree. I have raised the possibility of fashioning a group tree by bringing a small plastic or metal tree into the session and then inviting clients participating in the group to develop "leaves." I bring in paper of various colors and textures, scissors, various writing tools, paste, and many different kinds of materials that can be used to decorate the leaves that the clients make, such as beads, ribbons, and glitter in multiple colors. Clients can then create a leaf and write on their leaf a goal, a wish for their own future, or a resolution that reflects a change that they are committing to make. Each client is provided with string or yarn in order to hang the leaf on the tree. Clients are then invited to share with the other group members the significance of both their leaf and the process of creating their leaf.

Individuals in one group in which I utilized the metaphor of the tree in this manner used the opportunity to visualize their goals, to make new resolutions for change, and to reflect on the positive aspects of their lives. Several individuals wrote on their leaves, "Stop smoking," while others wrote, "Go to college," "Stay employed," and "I am thankful for life that the Man upstairs is providing for me." All of the clients indicated that they enjoyed using this metaphor because the exercise required that they reflect on and write down their goals, which renewed their hopes that they might achieve them; discuss their aspirations with other group members, which afforded them increased support in their efforts to achieve their goals; and think about the future, which helped them to believe that they might have one (in contrast to committing suicide or dying of a chronic illness).

REFERENCES

Austin, J., & Dankwort, J. C. (1994). Standards for batterer programs: A review and analysis. *Journal of Interpersonal Violence, 14*(2), 152–168.

Begley, C. E., Annegers, J. F., Swann, A. C., Lewis, C., Coan, S., Schnapp, L. B., et al. (2001). The lifetime cost of bipolar disorder in the US: An estimate for new cases in 1998. *Pharmacoeconomics, 19,* 483–495.

Bertalanffy, L. V. (1968). *General systems theory: Foundation, development, application.* New York: George Braziller.

Bloch, S., & Singh, B. S. (1997). *Understanding troubled minds: A guide to mental illness and its treatment.* Melbourne, Australia: Melbourne University Press.

Bybee, D., Mowbray, C. T., Oyserman, D., & Lewandowski, L. (2006). Variability in community functioning of mothers with serious mental illness. *Journal of Behavioral Health Services and Research, 30*(3), 269–289.

Catholic Culture. (2008). Jesse Tree. Last accessed February 22, 2008; Available at http://www.catholicculture.org/liturgicalyear/activities/view.cfm?id=956

Colom, F., Vieta, E., Tacci, M. J., Sanchez-Moreno, J., & Scott, J. (2005). Identifying and improving non-adherence in bipolar disorder. *Bipolar Disorders, 7*(5 Suppl), 24–31.

de Saint-Exupéry, A. (2002). *A guide for grown-ups: Essential wisdom from the collected works of Antoine de Saint-Exupéry.* San Diego, CA: Harcourt, Inc.

Dutton, D. G., & Golant, S. K. (1995). *The batterer: A psychological profile.* New York: Basic Books.

Elgood, H. (1999). *Hinduism and the religious arts.* London: Cassell.

Felder, R., & Victor, B. (1996). *Getting away with murder: Weapons for the war against domestic violence.* New York: Simon and Schuster.

Glynn, S. M., Cohen, A. M., Dixon, L. B., & Niv, N. (2006). The potential impact of the recovery movement on family interventions for schizophrenia: Opportunities and obstacles. *Schizophrenia Bulletin, 32*(3), 451–463.

Gondolf, E. W., & Russell, D. (1986). The case against anger control treatment programs for batterers. *Response, 9,* 2–5.

Hall, M. P. (2003). *The secret teachings of all ages: An encyclopedic outline of Masonic, Hermetic, Qabbalistic and Rosicrucian symbolical philosophy.* New York: Jeremy P. Tarcher/Penguin.

Ivey, A. E. (1998). Community genogram: Identifying strengths. In H. G. Rosenthal (Ed.), *Favorite counseling and therapy techniques: 51 therapists share their most creative strategies.* New York: Brunner-Routledge.

Iyengar, B. K. S. (2002). *The tree of yoga.* Boston: Shambala.

Johnson, S. L., Meyer, B., Winnett, C., & Small, J. (2000). Social support and self-esteem predict changes in bipolar depression but not mania. *Journal of Affective Disorders, 58(1),* 79–86.

Kirschenbaum, H., & Henderson, V. (Eds.). (1989). *The Carl Rogers reader.* Boston: Houghton Mifflin.

Lankevich, G. J. (2002). *The wit and wisdom of the Talmud: Proverbs, sayings, and parables for the ages.* Garden City Park, NY: Square One Classics.

Lieberman, J. A., Stroup, T. S., McEvoy, J. P., Swartz, M. S., Rosenheck, R. A., Perkins, D. O., et al. (2005). Effectiveness of antipsychotic drugs in patients with chronic schizophrenia. *New England Journal of Medicine, 353(12),* 1209–1223.

Lingam, R., & Scott, J. (2002). Treatment non-adherence in affective disorder. *Acta Psychiatrica Scandinavia, 105(3),* 164–172.

Maslow, A. H. (1970). *Motivation and personality* (2nd ed.). New York: Harper & Row.

Miklowitz, D. J., & Goldstein, M. J. (1990). Behavioral family treatment for patients with bipolar affective disorder. *Behavior Modification, 14,* 457–489.

Novak, P. (1994). *The world's wisdom: Sacred texts of the world's religions.* New York: HarperCollins.

Osterberg, L., & Blaschke, T. (2005). Adherence to medication. *New England Journal of Medicine, 353,* 487–497.

Perlick, D. A., Rosenheck, R. A., Kaczynski, R., & Kozma, L. (2004). Medication non-adherence in bipolar disorder: a patient-centered review of research findings. *Clinical Approaches in Bipolar Disorders, 3,* 56–64.

Pescosolido, B. A., Gardner, C. B., & Lubell, K. M. (1998). How people get into mental health services: stories of choice, coercion and "muddling through" from "first time." *Social Science & Medicine, 46(2),* 275–286.

Rigazio-DiGilio, S. A., Ivey, A. E., Kunkler-Peck, K. P., & Grady, L. T. (2005). *Community genograms: Using individual, family, and cultural narratives with clients.* New York: Teachers College Press.

Robbins, S. P., Chatterjee, P., & Canda, E. R. (1998). *Contemporary human behavior theory: A critical perspective for social work.* Boston: Allyn and Bacon.

Rogers, N. (2001). Person-centered expressive arts therapy: A path to wholeness. In Rubin, J. A. (Ed.), *Approaches to art therapy: Theory and technique* (pp. 163–177). New York: Brunner-Routledge.

Satir, V. (1964). *Conjoint family therapy.* Palo Alto, CA: Science and Behavior Books.

Satir, V. (1972). *Peoplemaking.* Palo Alto, CA: Science and Behavior Books.

Schumann, H. W. (1973). *Buddhism: An outline of its teachings and schools* (G. Feuerstein, Trans.). Wheaton, IL: Quest Books.

Smith, H. (1991). *The world's religions: Our great wisdom traditions.* San Francisco: HarperSanFrancisco.

Snelling, J. (1991). *The Buddhist handbook: A complete guide to Buddhist schools, teaching, practice, and history.* New York: Barnes & Noble Books.

Torrey, E. F., & Knable, M. B. (2002). *Surviving manic depression: A manual on bipolar disorder for patients, families and providers.* New York: Basic Books.

SUGGESTIONS FOR FURTHER READING

Tree of Knowledge: Good and Evil

Stein, M. (Ed.). (1995). *Jung on evil.* Princeton, NJ: Princeton University Press.

Zimbardo, P. (2007). *The Lucifer effect: Understanding how good people turn evil.* New York: Random House, Inc.

Tree of Nourishment: Relationships

Schwartz, R. C. (1995). *Internal family systems therapy.* New York: Guilford Press.

Walsh, F. (Ed.). (1999). *Spiritual resources in family therapy.* New York: Guilford Press.

Tree of Enchantment: Self-Actualization

Capacchione, L. (1988). *The power of your other hand: A course in channeling the inner wisdom of the right brain.* North Hollywood, CA: Newcastle Publishing Co., Inc.

Capacchione, L. (2000). *Visioning: Ten steps to designing the life of your dreams.* New York: Jeremy P. Tarcher/Putnam.

CHAPTER 11

Strengthening the Foundation:

Underlying Theory

THE PURPOSE OF METAPHOR

How is it that the use of metaphor in counseling can help clients? What is the basis for this approach?

The use of metaphor in therapy serves numerous purposes. First, metaphor allows both the therapist and the client to approach a situation indirectly, tactfully, and empathetically (Seiden, 2004). Perhaps a client is not quite ready to confront a particular situation or issue directly. The use of metaphor allows him or her to circumnavigate and contemplate the issue, without having to commit immediately to a particular stance, perspective, or resolution. And, because clients through the use of metaphor can narrow or widen the distance between themselves and the situation or issue with which they are dealing, they retain control over the depth and duration of their exploration. As an example, George had worked with the metaphor of the Yellow Brick Road for more than a year before he was able to acknowledge to himself that he was gay. Reliance on the metaphor allowed him to maintain a distance from that realization and gradually move closer to and farther from his Truth depending upon his level of comfort and the circumstances in his life outside the therapy room.

In this regard, it is important that you, as a skilled therapist, remain attuned to the client's response to a particular metaphor. You may want to merely suggest a specific metaphor, much as one might launch a small model sailboat on a lake and watch where the water and the wind choose to take it. This is the approach that I used with George in using the metaphor of the Yellow Brick Road. If I had incessantly forged ahead with the metaphor, much as the operator of a battery-powered toy motorboat on a still lake might race his boat to the opposite side in the least amount of time possible, I could have exacerbated George's level of anxiety, increased his defensiveness, and reduced the likelihood that he would have returned to the issues that were so troubling to him.

Because the metaphor permits the client to maintain distance from the quality, attribute, or situation that he or she is exploring, it also affords the client the opportunity to learn how to separate content from process. Consider, as an example, the bicycle metaphor. As individuals move forward in life, they get caught up in its content: what is happening to them, what they are doing at a particular moment—in essence, the stuff that constitutes the fabric of their lives. They are on their bicycle, paying attention to the pedaling. By using the metaphor of the bicycle, the clients can step back and view themselves on the bicycle; they can see where they have been and where they are now, and they can begin to get a sense of where it is that they would like to go; as they examine the content of their lives, they can develop a greater understanding of their own actions and the meaning of these actions. In other words, they can begin to respond to the situations they encounter, rather than merely reacting to them. They can see the forest *and* the trees along their path, and they can choose *how* they proceed down their path, whether it is by pedaling or with the roar of an engine.

Metaphor provides a mechanism for the creation of polyvocality, that is, the use of the client's interpersonal and social resources to expand the sources of input into the client's environment and experience (Gergen, 1999). You witness the client "unearthing" his or her strengths in the context of metaphor; your observation of these strengths validates their existence and contributes to the expansion of the client's view of himself or herself.

Consider, for instance, how the metaphors of the stone soup and the alphabet soup can be used in a group to effectuate this expansion. As described earlier in this volume, clients can be invited in the context of a group to enumerate one of their qualities for each letter of the alphabet ("alphabet soup") or identify what they believe they contribute to others in their environment. One variant of this exercise would be to ask group members to identify one or more positive contributions that another group member contributes to the "stone soup."

Metaphor also provides a tool by which the client and the therapist co-create a mutually comfortable and acknowledged language, a shorthand that allows them both to recognize immediately specific instances or events in time. For instance, a reference by Brenda to "Lamb Chop" recalls for both of us her enumeration of those qualities that she feels that she lacks and those she wishes to develop. And, because it is a co-creation of the client and therapist, rather than being devised by the therapist alone, clients can assume ownership and take their metaphors with them upon leaving therapy as a "stone in their pocket" that serves to remind them of where they have been, where they are going, and the strengths that they have to aid them on their journey. When Geoffrey begins to feel worthless, useless, incompetent, and the embodiment of all of the innumerable negative attributes that he could possibly imagine, the memory of his alphabet soup and the positive qualities it embodies helps to restrain him from plunging headlong into a dark tunnel of gloom and despair.

Metaphor allows you and the client together to monitor and assess changes in the client's self-image, perceptions of his or her situation, goals for the future, and behavior towards himself or herself and others. The process and content of the client's use of a particular metaphor and the meaning and significance that he or she ascribes to that metaphor may change over time, thereby providing an opportunity to reflect on how much the client has grown and the nature of that growth. It provides you, the therapist, with an additional tool to measure the client's growth, change in symptoms, and relations with others. The information that you gather from this additional tool can be integrated with data that you obtain from other measures and mechanisms for assessment, thereby maximizing the validity of your observations (Fennig, Craig, Lavelle, Kovasznay, & Bromet, 1994; Fennig, Craig, Tanenberg, Karant, & Bromet, 1994; Meyer, 1996; Perry, 1992; Pilkonis et al., 1995; Steiner, Tebes, Sledge, & Walker, 1995).

WHY DOES METAPHOR WORK?

Using a Strengths-Based Approach

You may have noticed that many of the metaphors that I use allow, and often invite, clients to focus on their strengths and abilities. This emphasis derives from a strengths-based approach to therapy. This approach rests on five assumptions: (1) All people and environments possess strengths that can be identified and harnessed to improve their quality of life; (2) a consistent emphasis on strengths fosters client motivation; (3) the identification of client strengths requires a process of collaborative discovery between the client and the therapist; (4) a focus on strengths reduces the likelihood that the client will be, or will feel that he or she is, blamed for the presenting situation; and (5) all environments contain resources that can be accessed and used (De Jong & Miller, 1995).

A strengths-based approach requires that therapists ask positive questions about how people can cope, how they meet challenges, and how they triumph in overcoming the difficulties that they face in their daily lives (Moxley, 1997). As indicated earlier, every question asked carries the potential to generate a possible version of a life (Epston, quoted in Cowley & Springen, 1995). It further requires that the therapist evaluate the client's strengths and weaknesses in the contexts in which they occur, as well as the strengths and weaknesses of their environments; this enables both the therapist and the client to identify strengths that the client may not even realize exist (Cowger, 1994; Moxley, 1997). In this regard, the strengths-based approach resembles the focus of positive psychology on client strengths in the context of situational demands (Aspinwall & Staudinger, 2003). (The relationship between a strengths-based approach and positive psychology is discussed in greater detail below.) This emphasis on strengths at both the individual and environmental levels provides a foundation for clients' development of enhanced personal and social empowerment, that is, an enhanced ability to determine the direction of their own lives and to play an important role in the shaping of their own environments (Cowger, 1994).

You may have also observed that, despite the clients' often serious mental illnesses diagnoses, I do not raise the issue of these diagnoses and their illness symptoms with the metaphors that I use. This is not to say that I avoid discussing them; indeed, it is critical that clients have an opportunity to explore in a safe space the meaning of their illness, their symptoms, and the impact and meaning of the diagnosis and the symptoms on their daily lives and their hopes for the future. However, we do not approach this discussion from the vantage point of reducing pathology but, instead, focus on the strengths that the client can bring to bear in addressing the challenges and difficulties engendered by the diagnosis.

The focus of the strengths-based perspective on client strengths in the context in which they manifest facilitates the use of this perspective across cultures. Consider, as an example, the quality of familism. *Familismo,* or familism, has been called one of the most important culture-specific values of Puerto Ricans. It has been defined as a cultural value that includes a strong identification and attachment of individuals with their nuclear and extended families, including "adopted" friends and family members (Bravo, 1989; Salgado de Snyder & Padilla, 1987), and strong feelings of loyalty, reciprocity, and a solidarity among members of the same family (Glazer & Moynihan, 1963). Familism consists of structural, attitudinal, and behavioral components. Structural familism refers to the spatial and social boundaries "within which behaviors occur and attitudes acquire meaning and are delineated by the presence or absence of nuclear and extended family members" (Valenzuela & Dornbusch, 1994, pp. 18–19). Attitudinal aspects include beliefs and attitudes regarding the family with respect to feelings of loyalty, solidarity, and reciprocity; the behavioral component refers to actions associated with those feelings (Triandis,

Marin, Betancourt, Lisanski, & Chang, 1982). It has been posited that the Hispanic family may play a singularly critical protective role because of its associated strong ties and high levels of mutual loyalty, solidarity, reliance and trust (*familismo*) (Marin & Marin, 1991). However, the effects of *familismo* may be mediated by acculturation level and place of birth (Gil, Vega, & Dimas, 1994; Sabogal, Marin, Otero-Sabogal, Marin, & Perez-Stable, 1987; Vega, Zimmerman, Warheit, Apospori, & Gil, 1993).

Suppose, now, that your client has a strong belief in the value of *familismo*. She has been referred to you for therapy following discharge from a hospitalization for major depression. Suppose further that she suffered sexual abuse as a child and is now the target of her husband's physical abuse. Disclosure and discussion of these circumstances may represent to her extreme disloyalty to the family and a breach of trust. However, helping her to acknowledge, honor, and move past these traumatic events may be critical to her recovery from her depression.

Reliance on a strengths-based perspective allows the therapist to explore with the client the positive nature of familism and the circumstances in which the client believes that strong loyalties are appropriate. The use of metaphor permits the client to begin to entertain the notion that loyalty to a family member may be misplaced in the absence of mutuality and in situations in which such loyalty may represent a threat to one's actual survival.

The grounding of a metaphor on a strengths-based approach is critical to its successful use in such a situation. Suppose, for instance, that I am using the bicycle metaphor with this particular client to explore where she has been and is going with her relationships. As she looks down her path, there may be an "Aha!" moment, an epiphany, at which time she recognizes her role in the selection of her abusive partners. She then visualizes her crash on her bicycle if she continues down this same path. The client cannot be left to leave your office with this as her final mental image from her session with you. This could lead to a continued rumination about her own shortcoming, resulting in a further diminution of her self-worth and self-esteem and a deepening of her depression. Indeed, research suggests that self-absorbed rumination may lead to adverse outcomes, including an increase in pessimistic thoughts and memories, decreased concentration and motivation, and difficulties with problem solving (Lyubomirsky & Tkach, 2004; Nolen-Hoeksema, 2003).

What you can begin to do at this point is to guide her attention to her strengths that she used to help her survive and move past these relationships and how she might use these strengths to fashion a more pleasant and easily navigable path for her future. A focus on her strengths and the positive emotions associated with the realization of her strengths may foster additional growth and encourage the further development of coping skills (Frederickson, 2001). And, depending upon the client's response to the bicycle metaphor at the moment of her "Aha!" realization, it may be advisable never again to raise that metaphor with her yourself, but to address it only if she were to raise it, because of the level of trauma or anxiety that would be associated with the recollection.

Positive Psychology

Here we see more clearly the relationship between a strengths-based approach and positive psychology, and how both of these perspectives are relevant to the use of metaphor. Positive psychology has been defined as "the study of the conditions and processes that contribute to the flourishing or optimal functioning of people, groups, and institutions" (Gable & Haidt, 2005). It seeks

> to catalyze a change in psychology from a preoccupation with repairing the worst things in life to also building the best qualities in life. . . . [W]e must bring the building of strength to the forefront in the treatment and prevention of mental illness (Seligman, 2002, p. 3).

Positive psychology operates at the subjective level of experience, such as feelings of past satisfaction, present feelings of joy, and positive thoughts about the future; at the individual level with respect to positive personal attributes, such as one's wisdom or ability to persevere; and at the group level, reflected in a movement towards better citizenship, as evidenced by civility and altruism (Gillham & Seligman, 1999; Seligman & Csikszentmihalyi, 2000). "Positive therapy," then, refers to any therapeutic approach that focuses on clients' strengths and positive attributes (Wong, 2006).

Accordingly, positive psychology considers the strengths and deficits of both the person and the environment (Wright & Lopez, 2002). A strengths-based approach represents a specific application of positive psychology (Wong, 2006), as do solution-focused therapy (de Shazer & Berg, 1992) and hope therapy (Lopez, Floyd, Ulven, & Snyder, 2000; Snyder, Rand, & Sigmon, 2002). Mental health is viewed as the corollary of mental illness and, like mental illness, reflects a constellation of symptoms (Keyes & Lopez, 2002). In contrast to mental illness, these are symptoms of well-being rather than symptoms of dysfunction.

Let us consider how a therapeutic approach premised on positive psychology might differ from one utilizing a more deficit-focused approach. Suppose we wished to foster increased resilience in a young child. A deficit- or risk-oriented approach might seek to prevent homelessness through the establishment of rental assistance programs, reduce neighborhood violence, and prevent child abuse through the establishment of parenting programs for individuals considered at high risk of becoming abusive. These strategies focus on what is lacking and attempt to eliminate the perceived void. In contrast, strategies premised on positive psychology might include the encouragement of already-existing mentoring relationships for children and support cultural traditions that provide children with the opportunity to develop strong emotional bonds, a sense of stability and familiarity, and a sense of self-pride.

Cognitive-Perceptual Theory

The use of metaphor in therapy also rests on cognitive-perceptual theory and the nature of memory. Cognitive-perceptual theory does not focus on how an individual learns but rather on what the individual has learned that he or she has retained the longest, as keys to understanding the individual's perceptions of self and the surrounding world (Bruhn, 1990). This theory is compatible both with Piaget's theory of cognitive development and Erik Erikson's stage model of human growth and development, referred to in earlier chapters (Bruhn, 1990).

The contribution of cognitive-perceptual theory is as follows. Memory is organized around content (what happened?), time (what time of year/at what age?), person (who was involved?), place (where did it occur?), activity (what were you doing?), mood (what were you feeling at the time?), and attitude (what did you think about it/believe?) (Bruhn, 1990). We see, then, that much of our memory is tied to concrete experiences, such as sights and sounds and places and persons (Pinker, 2007). Metaphor provides clients with a concrete image that is grounded in substance (for example, the tree), space (the snowflake), time (movement up the ladder), and causation (the bicycle), and that may consequently stimulate their memories of their experiences (cf. Pinker, 2007). We see, then, that the "essence of metaphor is understanding and experiencing one kind of thing [the client's experience] in terms of another [the proffered metaphor]" (Lakoff & Johnson, 1980, p. 5). And, because metaphors are so ubiquitous in our use of language, clients are able to relate to their use. Consider, for instance, the metaphors reflected by statements such as "His idea came to fruition" [ideas are plants]; "They have a sick relationship" [love is a patient]; and "He is crazy about her" [love is mental illness] (Lakoff & Johnson, 1980).

What the client remembers is likely selective, rather than photographic. Whether and how something is remembered largely depend on its utility, that is, the extent to which a major lesson about the self, others, or the world has been learned, and on adaptation, the extent to which the memory focuses on unresolved issues. However, the client may be unable to articulate clearly or even delineate his or her feelings or ideas; metaphor serves as a tool that facilitates both the identification and the communication of these abstractions.

REFERENCES

Aspinwall, L. G., & Staudinger, U. M. (2003). A psychology of human strengths: Some central issues of an emerging field. In L. G. Aspinwall & U. M. Staudinger (Eds.), *A psychology of human strengths: Fundamental questions and future directions for a positive psychology* (pp. 9–22). Washington, DC: APA Books.

Bravo, M. (1989). *Las redes de apoyo social y las situaciones de desastre: Estudio de la población adulta en P.R.* Rio Piedras, Puerto Rico: University of Puerto Rico.

Bruhn, A. R. (1990). Cognitive-perceptual theory and the projective use of autobiographical memory. *Journal of Personality Assessment, 55,* 95–114.

Cowger, C. D. (1994). Assessing client strengths: Clinical assessment for client empowerment. *Social Work, 39,* 262–268.

Cowley, G., & Springen, K. (1995, April 17). Rewriting life stories. *Newsweek,* 70–74.

De Jong, P., & Miller, S. D. (1995). How to interview for client strengths. *Social Work, 40,* 729–736.

de Shazer, S., & Berg, I. K. (1992). Doing therapy: A post-structural re-vision. *Journal of Marital and Family Therapy, 18,* 71–81.

Fennig, S., Craig, T. J., Lavelle, J., Kovasznay, B., & Bromet, E. J. (1994). Best-estimate versus structured interview-based diagnosis in first-admission psychosis. *Comprehensive Psychiatry, 35,* 341–348.

Fennig, S., Craig, T. J., Tanenberg-Karant, M., & Bromet, E. J. (1994). Comparison of facility and research diagnoses in first-admission psychotic patients. *American Journal of Psychiatry, 151,* 1423–1429.

Frederickson, B. L. (2001). The role of positive emotions in positive psychology: The broaden-and-build theory of positive emotions. *American Psychologist, 56,* 218–226.

Gable, S. L., & Haidt, J. (2005). What (and why) is positive psychology? *Review of General Psychology, 9,* 103–110.

Gergen, K. J. (1999). *An invitation to social construction.* London: Sage.

Gil, A. G., Vega, W. A., & Dimas, J. (1994). Acculturative stress and personal adjustment among Hispanic adolescent boys. *Journal of Community Psychology, 22,* 43–54.

Gillham, J. E., & Seligman, M. E. P. (1999). Footsteps on the road to positive psychology. *Behaviour Research and Therapy, 37,* S163–S173.

Glazer, N., & Moynihan, D. P. (1963). *Beyond the melting pot.* Cambridge, MA: Harvard-MIT Press.

Keyes, C. L. M., & Lopez, S. J. (2002). Toward a science of mental health: Positive directions in diagnosis and interventions. In C. R. Snyder & S. J. Lopez (Eds.), *Handbook of positive psychology* (pp. 45–59). New York: Oxford University Press.

Lakoff, G., & Johnson, M. (1980). *Metaphors we live by.* Chicago: University of Chicago Press.

Lopez, S. J., Floyd, R. K., Ulven, J. C., & Snyder, S. R. (2000). Hope therapy: Helping clients build a house of hope. In R. C. Snyder (Ed.), *Handbook of hope: Theory, measures, and interventions* (pp. 123–150). San Diego, California: Academic Press.

Lyubomirsky, S., & Tkach, C. (2004). The consequences of dysphoric rumination. In C. Papageorgiou & A. Wells (Eds.), *Rumination: Nature, theory, and treatment of negative thinking in depression* (pp. 21–41). Chichester, UK: Wiley.

Marin, G., & Marin, B. V. (1991). *Research with Hispanic populations.* Newbury Park, California: Sage Publications.

Meyer, G. J. (1996). The Rorschach and MMPI: Toward a more scientifically differentiated understanding of cross-method assessment. *Journal of Personality Assessment, 67,* 558–578.

Moxley, D. P. (1997). Clinical social work in psychiatric rehabilitation. In J. R. Brandell (Ed.), *Theory and practice in clinical social work* (pp. 618–661). New York: Free Press.

Nolen-Hoeksema, S. (2003). *Women who think too much: How to break free of overthinking and reclaim your life.* New York: Henry Holt.

Perry, J. C. (1992). Problems and considerations in the valid assessment of personality disorders. *American Journal of Psychiatry, 149,* 1645–1653.

Pilkonis, P. A., Heape, C. L., Proietti, J. M., Clark, S. W., McDavid, J. D., & Pitts, T. E. (1995). The reliability and validity of two structured diagnostic interviews for personality disorders. *Archives of General Psychiatry, 52,* 1025–1033.

Pinker, S. (2007). *The stuff of thought: Language as a window into human nature.* New York: Viking.

Sabogal, F., Marin, G., Otero-Sabogal, R., Marin, B. V., & Perez-Stable, E. J. (1987). Hispanic familism and acculturation: What changes and what doesn't. *Hispanic Journal of Behavioral Sciences, 9,* 397–412.

Salgado de Snyder, N., & Padilla, A. M. (1987). Social support networks: Their availability and effectiveness. In M. Gaviria & J. Arana (Eds.), *Health and behavior: Research agenda for Hispanics* (pp. 93–107). The Simón Bolívar Research Monograph Series No. 1. Chicago: University of Illinois at Chicago.

Seiden, H. M. (2004). On the "music of thought": The use of metaphor in poetry and psychoanalysis. *Psychoanalytic Psychology, 21,* 638–644.

Seligman, M. E. P. (2002). Positive psychology, positive prevention, and positive therapy. In C. R. Snyder & S. J. Lopez (Eds.), *Handbook of positive psychology* (pp. 3–9). New York: Oxford University Press.

Seligman, M. E. P., & Csikszentmihalyi, M. (2000). Positive psychology: An introduction. *American Psychologist, 55,* 5–14.

Snyder, C. R., Rand, K. L., & Sigmon, D. R. (2002). Hope theory: A member of the positive psychology family. In C. R. Snyder & S. J. Lopez (Eds.), *Handbook of positive psychology* (pp. 257–276). New York: Oxford University Press.

Steiner, J. L., Tebes, J. K., Sledge, W. H., & Walker, M. L. (1995). A comparison of the Structured Clinical Interview for *DSM-III-R* and clinical diagnoses. *Journal of Nervous and Mental Disease, 183,* 365–369.

Triandis, H. C., Marin, G., Betancourt, H., Lisanski, J., & Chang, B. (1982). *Dimensions of familism among Hispanic and mainstream Navy recruits.* Technical Report No. 14, Department of Psychology. Champaign: University of Illinois. Cited in F. I. Soriano. (1993). AIDS and intravenous drug use among Hispanics in the U.S.: Considerations for prevention efforts. In R. S. Mayers, B. L. Kail, & T. D. Watts (Eds.). *Hispanic Substance Abuse* (pp. 131–144). Springfield, IL: Charles C. Thomas.

Valenzuela, S. M., & Dornbusch, S. M. (1994). Familism and social capital in the academic achievement of Mexican origin and Anglo adolescents. *Social Science Quarterly, 75,* 18–36.

Vega, W. A., Zimmerman, R. S., Warheit, G. J., Apospori, E., & Gil, A. G. (1993). Risk factors for early adolescence drug use in racial/ethnic groups. *American Journal of Public Health, 83,* 185–189.

Wong, Y. J. (2006). The future of positive therapy. *Psychotherapy, Theory, Research, Practice, Training, 43,* 151–153.

Wright, B. A., & Lopez, S. J. (2002). Widening the diagnostic focus: A case for including human strengths and environmental resources. In C. R. Snyder & S. J. Lopez (Eds.), *Handbook of positive psychology* (pp. 26–44). New York: Oxford University Press.

SUGGESTIONS FOR FURTHER READING

Perception and Behavior

Combs, A. W., & Snygg, D. (1959). *Individual behavior: A perceptual approach to behavior.* New York: Harper & Row.

Damasio, A. (1994). *Descartes' error: Emotion, reason, and the human brain.* New York: Penguin Books.

Perception and Meaning

Blumer, H. (1969). *Symbolic interactionism: Perspective and method.* Berkeley: University of California Press.

Csordas, T. J. (Ed.). (1994). *Embodiment and experience: The existential ground of culture and self.* Cambridge, UK: Cambridge University Press.

Perception & Mental Well-Being

Siegel, D. J. (2007). *The mindful brain: Reflection and attunement in the cultivation of well-being.* New York: W. W. Norton & Company.

CHAPTER 12

Stepping Out From The Door:

How to Create and Use Metaphor for Healing, Growth, and Change

SOURCES OF METAPHOR

The sources of metaphor are almost limitless. They can be derived from religious texts, folk tales, songs, stories, and experiences of daily life. The use of metaphor and storytelling are frequently intertwined. While metaphors often serve as the basis for the development of stories or rituals, they may also be derived from stories. As such, they may serve as a shorthand to refer to shared events or knowledge (Johnson, 1995). I have found that metaphors are most successful across a wider range of persons when they embody and reflect a universal experience, such as a tree.

The following six objects drawn from common experience illustrate how metaphors can be formulated and then used in the context of counseling. Each object listed below has been paired with one or more goals that can serve as the focus for its use.

Train. The metaphor of the train can be used to help in the development of future direction, to emphasize the need for determination and perseverance, to explore potential difficulties in achieving one's goals, and as a mechanism for understanding one's interactions and relationships with others. It can also be used to explore the role that a client will play or the energy that he or she will devote to the attainment of a goal or objective. As an example, the train may have to go through valleys and up and around treacherous mountains to reach its intended station, just as the client may encounter seemingly insurmountable obstacles in working toward a goal. In any given situation, does the client perceive himself or herself as the engine, pulling the rest of the train (group); as the caboose, following where the other parts of the train go; or maybe the dining car, providing nourishment to others on the journey? Or does the client place himself or herself outside of the train as the conductor, as the ticketmaster, or as the engineer? Where the client situates himself or herself as part of the train metaphor may change over time as the context of his or her life changes, as he or she feels more or less mastery in life, and as he or she grows in self-understanding.

Onion. The metaphor of the onion can be used to examine the complexity or multiple layers of the client's being that must be known in order to achieve self-understanding. It can also be used as a vehicle for understanding relationship dynamics. For instance, clients may become frustrated with the arduous process of counseling, feeling that their work should be done sooner rather than later, wanting a quick fix to life's problems. The metaphor of the onion can be used as a way of helping them to understand, appreciate, and treasure their own complexity and the joy that comes from seeing and learning about the many layers of themselves that, as in an onion, each have their own unique texture and taste.

Cog. The metaphor of a cog in a wheel is an excellent one to help clients develop an understanding of their relationships and their place in their constellation of relationships. For those clients who prefer to know the theoretical basis of the metaphors that you introduce, the "cog in the wheel" is easily analogized to systems theory, which is premised on the idea that each individual plays a role within the larger system and that a change in the individual necessarily effectuates a change, even a small one, in the larger system of relationships. The client can be encouraged to examine the strength of each of the spokes that attaches to his or her wheel of relationships, his or her own strength as a cog on this wheel, and how well or poorly the wheel moves as a whole. Any number of questions can be posed using this metaphor:

- Are any of the spokes stronger or weaker than the others?
- What does that do to the balance of the wheel?
- How strong is this cog? What gives it its strength?
- In what way does the cog help the wheel function?
- Do you have/use these same qualities now? In what way?

Prism. The vision of a prism with its various facets and reflections of color provides the basis for an exploration of multiple perspectives in a given situation and the many options that may be available to a client who is trying to make a particular decision. Depending upon the angle from which a prism is viewed, the colors that are seen may be vastly different. Our affinity for that prism may depend on the color that we see. So, too, can one's response to a situation differ as a result of having a different perspective on the issue. Questions that can be asked of a client using this metaphor might include, depending on how the client uses the metaphor:

- Are there any colors in particular that reflect who you are?
- What qualities or parts of yourself do you think match those colors?
- Do you show different colors of yourself to different people in different situations? How do you decide which ones to show at any given time?
- Are there any parts of yourself or qualities that you have for which there are no colors in the prism? What qualities are those? What color(s) would you make them?

Mountains. Many clients may have heard the saying, "Don't make a mountain out of a molehill." The metaphor of the mountain can be used to help clients distinguish what is truly important (the mountain) from what is actually unimportant or superfluous to a given situation (the molehill). In this sense, it is useful in identifying priorities, in much the same way as the dough-nut metaphor ("Keep your eye on the doughnut, not the hole"). The metaphor can also be used to help clients visualize barriers and obstacles and how they might overcome them.

Puzzle. Successful completion of a jigsaw puzzle requires that the person completing the puzzle find just the right piece that fits with the pieces that are to surround it. The pieces must fit together both physically and with re-spect to their content and their color. This metaphor can be used to explore complementarity in relationships and roles. What strengths and weaknesses does each person bring to the relationship or situation that makes them or the situation a "good fit"? Do they build on and complement each other's strengths? Or do the weaknesses and limitations of each only serve to magnify those of the other? This metaphor may be especially helpful in working with clients who are experiencing conflict in their employment situations or their family or romantic relationships.

Clients may also offer metaphors when describing their situations, their illness, or the problems that they are facing. Michael White (2007, pp. 32–33) found that there is great diversity in the metaphors that clients themselves uti-lize. This diversity stems from the variety of their own experiences such as the equine world ("harnessing the problem"), the maritime world ("salvaging" one's life from the problem), geography ("reclaiming" life's territory from the prob-lem), and climate ("becoming deacclimated to the problem"), among others.

USING METAPHOR WITH CLIENTS

Introducing Metaphor to Your Clients

How to introduce metaphor into your work with clients and obtain cli-ent "buy-in" to working with this technique is likely to be one of the more difficult issues for counselors and therapists. It is important to recognize and acknowledge at the outset that some clients may be unwilling even to engage in the use of metaphor. Others may be hesitant, feeling that they will look silly to you or that it is for children.

I have found it helpful to approach the initial trial of metaphor by asking the client, "Are you willing to try an experiment with me?" Some clients will respond with, "Sure," at which point I can follow up with a specific metaphor that I think may be helpful.

Other clients may answer, "What do you mean, an experiment? What's going to happen?" or, alternatively, "What are you going to do with me?" I respond by explaining that I have found that using metaphor helps many people because holding an image in one's mind may make it easier to talk about something or to visualize a situation or recall a feeling. I also explain that it is an experiment, and that "experiment" means that it is something that we can try, but that we do not know whether it will work or not work. I do not use the word "fail." And, because we cannot know ahead of time whether an experiment will work or not, which makes it an experiment, the client is relieved of the responsibility for making sure it works or the shame or embarrassment if it should fail. There simply is no failure because it was an experiment to begin with. I also point out that sometimes a certain metaphor might not work, whereas another might seem more relevant to a particular client. If the client finds that a particular metaphor is not help-ful, I explain, we can always try another one at some indefinite time in the future if the client is interested in doing so. In my experience, most clients are willing to try metaphor based on this explanation because there is no risk of failure.

Which Clients Can Benefit?

Some mental health professionals have responded in disbelief when I have told them of my use of metaphor with individuals who have thought disor-ders, such as schizophrenia, and mood disorders, such as bipolar disorder or major depression. They have questioned, for instance, the ability of someone with schizophrenia to relate a metaphor to his or her own situation, or the ability of someone with bipolar disorder to reframe his or her perception of his or her own behavior through the use of a metaphor.

I have found, however, that both clients with serious mood disorders and those with thought disorders are able to utilize metaphors as a way of exploring their past and current situations, their self-concept, their relation-ships, and their hopes and fears. Because metaphor utilizes familiar, concrete images that may provoke few feelings of threat or vulnerability, the integration of metaphor as a technique into therapeutic modalities may allow clients to initiate their exploration of such critical issues more effectively.

As with every therapeutic approach and technique, metaphors will not be helpful to all clients. In general, I have found that my use of metaphor has not been beneficial for two groups of individuals. The first consists of those who are intellectually limited, such as individuals with mental retardation. Although they are able to describe the subject of the metaphor, such as a tree or snowflake, they are unable to relate the characteristics of that object to themselves because of the limitations of their intellectual functioning.

The second group of clients with whom I have found metaphor to be unhelpful consists of women in their early adult years who are experiencing considerable conflict in their relationships with their mothers. I have not examined the issue systematically, but it appears my use of metaphor with them may be reminiscent of storytelling by their mothers and, as such, may be perceived as a threat to their attempts to separate themselves from their mothers. This response may be more pronounced in their work with me because I am female and am at an age that approximates that of their mothers, thereby raising significant transference issues.

Sometimes clients may not respond to a metaphor directly, but the use of the metaphor may prompt the client to view his or her situation with greater insight or clarity. This was the case with Phoebe, a client whom I was seeing on an individual basis. Phoebe was an African American woman in her mid-twenties who began seeing me following the termination of her employment and the break-up of her romantic relationship.

When Phoebe and I first started our work together, she indicated that she had never thought of her own strengths, despite the many obstacles that she had encountered and had had to overcome somehow. Phoebe had been subjected to severe sexual abuse as a young girl and, as a result, had become quite depressed. When she attempted to enlist her mother's protection against the family member who had done this to her, her mother had become enraged, had accused her of lying, and had beaten her. Finally, at the school's urging, Phoebe's mother had allowed her to see a social worker for counseling. In response to her mother's demand of the social worker that she be told what Phoebe had said during the session, the social worker explained that communications between a client and therapist are confidential. Phoebe's mother became furious, refused to allow Phoebe to continue in counseling, and evicted her from the household.

Phoebe remains depressed about her "lack of a family foundation," as she puts it. She has rarely had any contact with her mother or siblings since her mother ejected her, approximately 10 years ago. Since that time, she has lived, in her words, "from couch to couch," staying with various friends, the families of various friends, or various romantic partners. She completed her GED and continues to dream of going to college one day and becoming a famous writer. She has held a variety of part-time temporary jobs with various agencies and companies, but would like to find employment that would allow her to become financially independent. Phoebe was fired from her last three places of employment, once for "slacking off," once for using marijuana (which she claims was a "bogus" charge), and once because of her sexual orientation, which favors both men and women.

I asked Phoebe how she had coped with all of the stresses and difficulties that she had encountered. "Mostly blunts [marijuana rolled in a cigar with the tobacco removed] and alcohol," she informed me. Phoebe was initially unable to explain how she had coped apart from using these substances. We utilized the metaphor of the tree to help her identify the strengths that she had and that she could develop even further to help her cope with stress and reach her goals. Phoebe didn't frame her response as if she were a tree. However, it can be seen that the idea of a tree and its germination was embedded in her response ("The good seeds were sowed in my younger years") and may have helped her to identify her strengths and the elements of her life that provided her with a greater sense of stability and security—in other words, spiritual and emotional nourishment:

> "If you think of yourself as a tree, with a trunk and roots, and branches, and leaves, what would those be?"
>
> "I have the gift of intelligence and insight. It is also a curse because even though I see what I do, I can't get out of my self-destructive cycle. I feel like I will never change. I need to stay focused. Only by the grace of God. The good seeds were sowed in my younger years. I always dreamed of making it big, of being on a pedestal, holding onto that dream and knowing that it can come true, helping people keep from making my mistakes. Trying to make my grandmother proud. It's my relation with God, really, that gives me my strength, that grounds me. I wonder sometimes if God really, really loves me, if He hears me."

When used in the context of group work or family counseling, metaphors may help to develop and strengthen bonds, reinforce a sense of safety and refuge, and define boundaries. Metaphors such as the alphabet soup and the stone soup, when used in a group, create an opportunity for group members to validate each other's positive contributions, while still acknowledging the pain and difficulties that each is experiencing.

Selecting the Metaphor

The counselor's or therapist's selection of an appropriate metaphor depends on several factors: (1) the goal of the particular session; (2) what has been accomplished in previous sessions, if any; (3) the client's familiarity with specific objects; and (4) the therapeutic orientation of the therapist. Although a specific metaphor can be used for a variety of purposes, such as demonstrated by "The Tree," certain metaphors lend themselves more easily to the achievement of specific goals. A session devoted to the development of future goals is more likely to be successful in initiating that process if the metaphor that is used implies future direction, such as "The Bicycle." The use of a metaphor such as "The Snowflake" is unlikely to have any meaning or significance to a client who has never seen snow; in such a situation, the transformation of the metaphor into a more recognizable object, such as a cloud or water drop or other familiar object, is advisable. Finally, both the selection of the metaphor and how the client's response to the metaphor is interpreted will necessarily depend upon the therapist's own theoretical perspective.

The same metaphor can be utilized multiple times during the course of longer-term counseling or therapy. The repetition of the same metaphor may help both the client and the therapist identify critical changes that have occurred and areas or domains that require further attention. For instance, the river metaphor can be utilized at multiple points in time to identify the changes that the client has undergone and the abilities and skills that he or she has utilized in order to move forward productively. It can also be used to examine changes in the larger context of the client's life, as the client confronts new and different obstacles, challenges, and adventures. For example, perhaps there are new stones in the river bed, or sudden changes in the velocity of the river, or an unexpected waterfall, or the construction of a dam. The client's periodic use of the tree metaphor may reveal changes in the "root" system from which the client derives support, the relationship between the leaves or other persons in the client's world, transformations in the colors (temperament) of the leaves, or the strength, texture, and height of the trunk, that is, the client's core identity.

INTEGRATING METAPHOR INTO CONVENTIONAL MODALITIES

Art Therapy

The use of metaphor in conjunction with art therapy was discussed briefly in "The Tree." Like metaphor, art therapy can utilize or be integrated into any of various orientations within psychology and psychotherapy, including a psychoanalytic approach derived from Freud; a Jungian analytic approach; a humanistic approach derived from phenomenology, Gestalt therapy, or other humanistic perspectives; and a behavioral or psycho-educational approach, such as cognitive-behavioral therapy (Rubin, 2001). This complexity and diversity prohibits an examination of how metaphor can be integrated into each such approach with art therapy within the scope of this chapter. Accordingly, this section focuses on the use of the river metaphor to illustrate how one metaphor can be integrated into solution-focused therapy with an individual client.

Solution-focused therapy is premised on the mutual development of goals by the therapist and the client. Therapists employing this approach attempt to "1) change 'the doing' of the situation that is perceived as problematic; 2) change the 'viewing' of the situation that is perceived as problematic; and 3) evoke resources, solutions, and strengths to bring to the situation that is problematic" (O'Hanlon & Weiner-Davis, 1989, pp. 126–127).

Suppose, for example, that a client is having difficulty with his relationships in the workplace and believes that his ineffectiveness is due to the micromanaging behavior of his supervisor. For a variety of reasons he wishes to find a way to address the situation, rather than searching for other employment. Relying on the use of the river metaphor, the client might draw a picture of the river with a huge dam in it, preventing the river from flowing downhill. The therapist could inquire into the accuracy of the client's observation that none of the water actually flows beyond the dam. This may stimulate an examination of what the client actually is able to accomplish, despite this seeming impediment, thereby changing the "doing." Next, the therapist may work with the client to identify those times when the water is able to flow beyond the dam, that is, when the client was able to be effective despite the supervisor, and the qualities of those situations that may have permitted or facilitated this success (the "viewing"). Finally, the client and therapist can focus on the identification of the client's inner strengths and resources that enabled him to be effective. Following this exploration, the therapist may ask the client to draw a picture of the river and compare this drawing to the previous one. The client can describe any changes in his depiction of the river and the relationship of any such changes to his new view of the situation.

Cognitive Behavioral Therapy

There are numerous cognitive-behavioral therapies, such as cognitive behavior modification (Meichenbaum, 1977), integrated cognitive behavior therapy (Wessler, 1984), and rational behavior training (Maultsby, 1984), among others. Because each therapeutic modality possesses unique characteristics, it is impossible to examine the use of metaphor in the context of each specific approach. Instead, we focus here on the characteristics that are common across the various approaches and the use of metaphor in this context.

Cognitive behavioral therapy (CBT) focuses on the client's thoughts, decisions, and values (the cognitive content) (Ingram & Kendall, 1986); the process by which the client selects and recalls information; the client's organization of the information that is received; and the client's underlying assumptions and beliefs, which serve as filters for screening and evaluating information from the environment (Rush & Beck, 1978). CBT encourages the client to examine a specific event of concern, the client's beliefs about that event, and his or her responses to the event, which derive from those beliefs (Ellis, 1991). CBT is premised on the assumption that the client's response to a given situation derives from irrational beliefs. Albert Ellis (1994) asserted that individuals in our society have been inculcated with 11 major irrational beliefs which, although frequently self-defeating, may serve as the "rationale" for our behavior:

1. Adults must be loved or accepted by all significant other individuals in their community.
2. One is inadequate and worthless unless one is competent and achieving in all important domains.
3. Individuals are their actions; if they behave badly, they are bad people.
4. Life is horrible and terrible when things don't go the way we would like or how we had planned.
5. Individuals have little or no ability to change the way that they feel or how they respond, because emotional disturbance is the result of external forces.
6. One should focus on issues or events that are potentially dangerous or worrisome.
7. It is not possible to confront and address one's responsibilities and difficulties in life; it is better to avoid them.
8. Individuals should be dependent on others to help them run their lives; they cannot do it on their own.
9. An individual's present behavior is determined by his or her past history, which will exert an influence on him or her into the indefinite future.
10. Others' disturbances are terrible, and one should be upset about them.
11. There is one correct solution to all human problems, and the failure to find the perfect solution is a terrible shortcoming.

A primary goal, then, is to assist the client through cognitive restructuring to recognize the irrational premise that underlies his or her response and to replace the irrationality with rationality, thereby leading to modification of the client's behavioral response.

Cognitive behavioral therapy represents a collaborative effort by the therapist and the client to resolve the client's problem. The therapist or counselor provides the client with information about the nature of the illness, intervention strategies, and tools by which to assess the success of the interventions. The client provides the content for the sessions, which consists of the client's views of himself or herself and others and his or her relations with others in the world. The approach to the identification and resolution of the problem is structured and often involves didactic instruction, homework assignments, guided discovery or questioning of the client, and the development of relapse prevention strategies.

Metaphor can be utilized in conjunction with the techniques of cognitive-behavioral therapy. For example, the metaphor of the elephant and the blind men can be utilized to examine the various ways of viewing a particular situation or potential responses to a given event or circumstance. Each of the blind men may represent a faulty assumption that underlies the client's response to a situation (the elephant). Replacement of each blind man with a rational "seeing" man will permit the client to see the entire elephant (situation) as it actually is and respond appropriately.

Consider the following example. Your client is upset because someone in her office failed to respond to her cheerful "Good morning" greeting. Her immediate (faulty) assumption is they the individual failed to greet her because he hates her. Her response, however, is akin to seeing only one part, perhaps the ear, of the elephant. It is critical that she understand that there is a larger elephant there in addition to the ear; other aspects of that elephant may challenge her underlying faulty assumption. This encourages her to search for alternative explanations for the failure of the individual to return her greeting; each such explanation, in essence, constitutes a different part of the elephant. The more explanations she can identify, the more of the actual elephant she is seeing. In this situation, other explanations (parts of the elephant) may be that the individual was having bad day, that the individual was preoccupied and didn't hear her, that the individual was late for a meeting or appointment and didn't want to stop, or the person was listening intently to a telephone conversation on a Bluetooth device that your client didn't see.

Dialectical Behavior Therapy

Unlike cognitive-behavioral therapy, which is premised on the assumption that it is irrational thinking or beliefs that serve as the basis for the client's emotional and behavioral response to an event or situation, dialectical behavior therapy (DBT) assumes that clients' perceptions of their experiences are generally accurate and that faulty perceptions do not play a major role in the development or prolongation of emotional pain (Marra, 2005). Rather, DBT emphasizes the emotions as the causative factor in the development of psychopathology, noting that clients' attempts to avoid and escape their emotions often paradoxically result in the intensification of the emotions' effects. In contrast, DBT asserts, acceptance of the pain will result in its diminution. DBT exercises are provided to assist the client in the development of mindfulness, interpersonal effectiveness, emotion regulation, and distress tolerance (McKay, Wood, & Brantley, 2007). Metaphors can often be used in conjunction with these exercises.

Consider the following example. A client may become quite upset in response to a difficult or unwanted situation. Rather than becoming increasingly angry, which may result in an increase in emotional pain (Greenwood, Thurston, Rumble, Waters, & Keefe, 2003), therapists utilizing DBT may advise their clients to engage in "radical acceptance," that is, to acknowledge their current situation without judging themselves or the situation itself (McKay et al., 2007). In this way, the client will be more likely to understand the details of the situation and the various approaches that can be utilized in response. Clients may be instructed to formulate "radical acceptance coping statements" to facilitate this process of acceptance (McKay et al., 2007).

One such radical acceptance coping statement is "Fighting the past only blinds me to my present" (McKay et al., 2007, p. 11). The bicycle metaphor could be utilized in conjunction with this radical acceptance coping statement to help clients explore what they are fighting about the past and how it is preventing them from seeing where they currently are on their bicycle. An alternative metaphor that could be used is that of Venetian blinds or a curtain; what is it that the client is blind to? What color/texture/thickness/width are those blinds/curtains? How can they be pulled aside? Should they be opened gradually or all at once? What will happen if/when they are opened? Who should open them?

Dialectical behavior therapy also teaches individuals to distract themselves from their pain by focusing on someone else (McKay et al., 2007). This exercise can be combined with the metaphor of the stone soup to identify with the client his or her qualities and skills that can be utilized in the process of doing something for someone else.

Narrative Therapy

Not infrequently, the stories that individuals tell about themselves are disempowering, reflecting the client's sense that he or she has lost agency in his or her own life. The use of narrative therapy allows the client to identify alternative stories that reflect his or her agency or empowerment; this reframing is known as repositioning or reclaiming the voice of the client. This approach has been analogized to consciousness-raising (Drewery & Winslade, 1997). The therapist is charged with the task of active listening in order to identify conflicting stories and hidden meanings ("deconstruction"), which can then be utilized by the client to identify underlying assumptions and differing interpretations.

Narrative therapy also makes use of externalizing conversations to move the discussion away from the client's ownership of "the problem" and associated guilt, blame, judgment, and recriminations and focus it, instead, on the exploration of the various dimensions of the client's situation (Monk, 1997). This approach recognizes that different "stories are possible, even about the same events. How we talk about it depends on our starting point, and how we explain what happens to us depends on the questions we ask" (Drewery & Winslade, 1997, p. 40).

As indicated previously, clients will often utilize metaphors derived from their own experiences in externalizing their problem or relating their story (White, 2007). However, the therapist can also utilize metaphors to assist clients in the process of reframing their story. As an example, the metaphor of the elephant and the blind men can be used as a vehicle for explaining the basis of narrative therapy, that is, the idea that even the same story may differ depending upon the starting point.

FUTURE DIRECTIONS

Important questions have yet to be answered. With which clients is the use of metaphor most acceptable? Most effective? Is the utilization of metaphor more likely to be effective with clients having certain diagnoses? Having cultural or religious heritages that utilize storytelling or metaphor as a vehicle for teaching? My work with metaphor has been exclusively with adults, from the age of 18 upwards. Although the clinical use of storytelling and metaphor with children has been examined in the literature (Costantino, Malgady, & Rogler, 1986; Gardner, 1993; Malgady, Rogler, & Costantino, 1990), relatively little research has rigorously evaluated the efficacy and effectiveness of this approach with youngsters and adolescents.

Is there a particular therapeutic approach that is most amenable to the integration of metaphor and that is most likely to achieve a positive outcome? It has been suggested that change in all forms of psychotherapy requires a good alliance between the client and the therapist (Bordin, 1979), which itself is dependent upon the degree of agreement that exists between the therapist and the client regarding the tasks and goals of the therapy and the quality of the relational bond between them. These three components—the tasks, the goals and the bond—mutually influence and inform each other. As has been stated,

> the *actual* effect of any particular intervention with a client is *always* determined by the client, not the therapist. The intentions and consequent actions of the therapist only trigger a response; they never determine it (Tomm, 1987, pp. 4–5) (emphasis in original).

Regardless of the therapeutic modality utilized, it is the quality of the therapeutic alliance that has been found to be most strongly associated with the outcome of psychotherapy (Gelso & Carter, 1994; Horvath & Symonds, 2001). Is this also true of the use of metaphor, that it is the therapeutic alliance that will be most determinative of the outcome?

REFERENCES

Bordin, E. S. (1979). The generalizability of the psychoanalytic concept of the working alliance. *Psychotherapy, 16,* 252–260.

Costantino, G., Malgady, R. G., & Rogler, L. H. (1986). Cuento therapy: A culturally sensitive modality for Puerto Rican children. *Journal of Consulting and Clinical Psychology, 54,* 639–645.

Drewery, W., & Winslade, J. (1997). The theoretical story of narrative therapy. In G. Monk, G. Winslade, K. Crocket, & D. Epston (Eds.), *Narrative therapy in practice: The archaeology of hope* (pp. 32–52). San Francisco: Jossey-Bass.

Ellis, A. (1991). The revised ABC's of rational-emotive therapy (RET). *Journal of Rational-Emotive and Cognitive-Behavior Therapy, 9*(3), 139–172.

Ellis, A. (1994). *Reason and emotion in psychotherapy: A comprehensive method of treating human disturbances* (rev. ed.). Secaucus, NJ: Birch Lane Press.

Gardner, R. A. (1993). *Storytelling in psychotherapy with children.* Northvale, NJ: Jason Aronson Inc.

Gelso, C., & Carter, J. (1994). Components of the psychotherapy relationship: Their interaction and unfolding during treatment. *Journal of Counseling Psychology, 41,* 296–306.

Greenwood, K. A., Thurston, R., Rumble, M., Waters, S. J., & Keefe, F. J. (2003). Anger and persistent pain: Current status and future directions. *Pain, 103,* 1–5.

Horvath, A., & Symonds, D. (1991). Relation between the working alliance and outcome in psychotherapy: A meta-analysis. *Journal of Counseling Psychology, 38,* 139–149.

Ingram, R. E., & Kendall, P. C. (1986). Cognitive clinical psychology: Implications of an information processing perspective. In R. E. Ingram (Ed.), *Information processing approaches to clinical psychology* (pp. 4–21). New York: Academic Press.

Johnson, A. C. (1995). Resiliency mechanisms in culturally diverse families. *The Family Journal: Counseling and Therapy for Couples and Families, 3(4)*, 316–324.

Malgady, R. G., Rogler, L. H., & Costantino, G. (1990). Hero/heroine modeling for Puerto Rican adolescents: A preventive mental health intervention. *Journal of Consulting and Clinical Psychology, 58*, 469–474.

Marra, T. (2005). *Dialectical behavior therapy in private practice: A practical and comprehensive guide.* Oakland, CA: New Harbinger Publications, Inc.

Maultsby, M. C. (1984). *Rational behavior therapy.* Englewood Cliffs, NJ: Prentice Hall.

McKay, M., Wood, J. C., & Brantley, J. (2007). *The dialectical behavior therapy skills workbook: Practical DBT exercises for learning mindfulness, interpersonal effectiveness, emotion regulation, and distress tolerance.* Oakland, CA: New Harbinger Publications, Inc.

Meichenbaum, D. (1977). *Cognitive-behavior modification.* New York: Plenum Press.

Monk, G. (1997). How narrative therapy works. In G. Monk, G. Winslade, K. Crocket, & D. Epston (Eds.), *Narrative therapy in practice: The archaeology of hope* (pp. 3–31). San Francisco: Jossey-Bass.

O'Hanlon, W., & Weiner-Davis, M. (1989). *In search of solutions: A new direction in psychotherapy.* New York: Norton.

Rubin, J. A. (2001). *Approaches to art therapy: Theory and technique* (2nd ed.). New York: Brunner-Routledge.

Rush, A. J., & Beck, A. T. (1978). Adults with affective disorders. In M. Hersen & A. S. Bellack (Eds.), *Behavior therapy in the psychiatric setting* (pp. 286–330). Baltimore: Williams & Wilkins.

Tomm, K. (1987). Interventive interviewing: Part I. Strategizing as a fourth guideline for the therapist. *Family Process, 26*, 3–13.

Wessler, R. L. (1984). Alternative conceptions of rational-emotive therapy: Toward a philosophically neutral psychotherapy. In M. A. Reda & M. J. Mahoney (Eds.), *The cognitive psychotherapies: Recent developments in theory, research, and practice* (pp. 65–79). Cambridge, MA: Ballinger.

White, M. (2007). *Maps of narrative practice.* New York: W. W. Norton & Company.

SUGGESTIONS FOR FURTHER READING

Sources of Metaphor

De Saint-Exupéry, A. (2000). *The little prince.* San Diego, CA: Harcourt, Inc.

Muth, J. J. (2005). *Zen shorts.* New York: Scholastic Press.

Schram, P. (1998). *Ten classic Jewish children's stories.* New York: Pitspopany.

Tatar, M. (Ed.). (2004). *The annotated brothers Grimm.* New York: W. W. Norton & Company.

Therapeutic Perspectives and Techniques

Beck, A. T. (1976). *Cognitive therapy and the emotional disorders.* New York: Penguin Books.

Orsillo, S. M., & Roemer, L. (Eds.). (2005). *Acceptance and mindfulness-based approaches to anxiety: Conceptualization and treatment.* New York: Springer.

Rubin, J. A. (2005). *Artful therapy.* New York: John Wiley & Sons, Inc.

Postscript

A number of the men and women mentioned in this volume with whom I worked on an individual basis have periodically contacted me to inform me of their progress. A few continue to see me on an individual basis for counseling, although more intermittently than before. Some of these individuals have made significant strides in dealing with their illnesses and their approach to life's difficulties, while others have not. As can be seen, as with any other therapeutic modality, the use of metaphor is not a panacea. For some, however, it has provided them with a new avenue for their journey.

Geoffrey is currently employed with a large-size company in his city of residence. He continues to follow his medication regimen faithfully. He has become increasingly healthy, both mentally and physically. As he has done so, his siblings have become more hostile towards him, which has prompted him to acknowledge the high level of dysfunction that exists in his family of origin. He has ceased all contact with his siblings because of their reactivity and unwillingness to allow him his independence, despite his stable mental health and high level of responsibility. He has expanded his network of friendships, which operate at varying levels of emotional depth and support. He has become financially secure and remains optimistic, albeit somewhat apprehensive, about his future.

Joseph stopped taking his medication several months prior to the completion of this volume, complaining that it makes him feel "flat." He has refused to consider other medications. He has recently been experiencing brief periods of depression and increasing difficulty in concentrating. He has been able to maintain steady employment and remains in college. However, his academic standing is tenuous because of frequent absences from his classes. He continues to live with his grandmother and has been making some effort to explore with his uncle his motivations for having abused Joseph sexually. He recently disclosed his homosexuality to a wider circle of acquaintances. After doing so, he expressed his relief, stating, "I feel like I don't have a monkey on my back any more."

Margaret's continued refusal to acknowledge her illness and to seek treatment culminated in another suicide attempt. Following a rather lengthy period of hospitalization, she began to adhere to a regimen of medication and therapy. Although she is now willing to venture more frequently outside of her familiar environment, she continues to believe that her current dissatisfaction with her life and the people around her stems from others' hostility towards her and their attempts to undermine her efforts and precipitate her failure.

Douglas was recently dismissed by his employer for insubordination and violation of company policy. Douglas acknowledges that he has had similar interactions with every employer for whom he has worked, but denies any role in such events. Instead, he attributes his work-related difficulties and repeated confrontations with supervisors to their "idiocy." He refuses to examine his own underlying issues that he projects into every encounter with someone in authority.

Joshua appears to have ceased all cutting and purging behaviors. He is attending a private university and is doing well academically.

Katy has continued to deny that she has bipolar disorder and refuses to seek care despite the efforts of her family members to convince her to seek treatment. She was terminated from employment as a result of her escalating aggressiveness and threatening behavior.

Tamara's girlfriend ended their year-long relationship, indicating that she needed space while Tamara "gets it together." Tamara did not adhere to the budget that they had developed together to pay Tamara's fine. As a result, she was sentenced to several days in jail in lieu of paying the fine. She is currently seeking employment.

Leon relocated to another major city and has secured employment as a youth counselor. He has completed his undergraduate degree and is seeking admission to graduate school on a part-time basis. He has been successful in having several pieces of his writing accepted for publication.

Index

SPRINGER PUBLISHING COMPANY

Using Superheroes in Counseling and Play Therapy

Lawrence C. Rubin, PhD, LMHC, RPT-S, Editor

"There is something democratic about a therapy that can respond empathically to the experiences that patients enjoy and feel that they understand emotionally."
—From the Foreword by **John Shelton Lawrence, PhD**
Morningside College, Emeritus

With an incisive historical foreword by John Shelton Lawrence and insight from contributors such as Michael Brody, Patty Scanlon, and Roger Kaufman, Lawrence Rubin takes us on a dynamic tour of the benefits of using these icons of popular culture and fantasy in counseling and play therapy. Not only can superheroes assist in clinical work with children, but Rubin demonstrates how they can facilitate growth and change with teens and adults. Early childhood memories of how we felt pretending to have the power to save the world or our families in the face of impending danger still resonate in our adult lives, making the use of superheroes attractive as well to the creative counselor.

In presenting case studies and wisdom gleaned from practicing therapists' experience, the book shows how it is possible to uncover children's secret identities, assist treatment of adolescents with sexual behavior problems, and inspire the journey of individuation for gay and lesbian clients, all by paying attention to our intrinsic social need for superhero fantasy and play.

List of Contributors:

Leya Barrett
Michael Brody
Jan Burte
George Enfield
Roger Kaufman
John Shelton Lawrence

Harry Livesay
William McNulty
Cory A. Nelson
Jeff Pickens
Robert Poole
Robert J. Porter

Karen Robertie
Lawrence C. Rubin
Jennifer Mendoza Sayers
Patty Scanlon
Ryan Weidenbenner
Carmela Wenger

2007 · 368 pp · Hardcover · 978-0-8261-0269-0

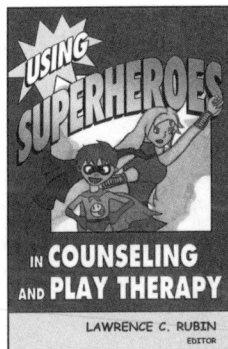

11 West 42nd Street, New York, NY 10036-8002 • Fax: 212-941-7842
Order Toll-Free: 877-687-7476 • Order Online: www.springerpub.com

Structured Group Psychotherapy for Bipolar Disorder

The Life Goals Program, Second Edition

Mark S. Bauer, MD, and **Linda McBride,** MSN

"The Life Goals Program...offers a comprehensive, empowering program that keeps the needs of the whole person at the center of treatment. It's refreshing to see a wellness-based model that links both medication and psychotherapy in such a logical and sensitive way. The Life Goals Program empowers us to seek wellness based on those issues that are of the highest importance to us."

Structured Group Psychotherapy for Bipolar Disorder

The Life Goals Program

Second Edition

Mark S. Bauer
Linda McBride

Springer Publishing Company

—**Sue Bergeson,** Deputy Executive Director
Depression and Bipolar Support Alliance (formerly National DMDA)

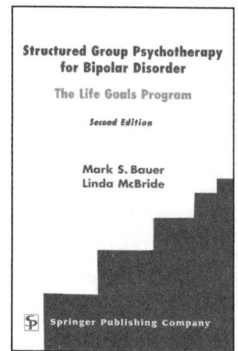

"The first edition...has been a central part of our research program to improve care for people with bipolar disorder. The second edition improves significantly on the first with expanded and updated educational information, a more user-friendly format for group leaders, and more emphasis on collaboration long-term treatment planning."

—**Gregory Simon,** MD, MPH
Investigator, Center for Health Studies, Group Health Cooperative

This updated and substantially revised edition not only incorporates the expansion of the pharmacological armamentarium available for treatment but also integrates the explosion of evidence-based data for psychosocial interventions. The authors, a psychiatrist-nurse team, have fine-tuned their two-phase treatment program and present a clear and concise approach to improving illness self-management skills, as well as social and occupational functioning.

2003 · 400 pp · Hardcover · 978-0-8261-1694-9

11 West 42nd Street, New York, NY 10036-8002 • **Fax: 212-941-7842**
Order Toll-Free: 877-687-7476 • **Order Online: www.springerpub.com**

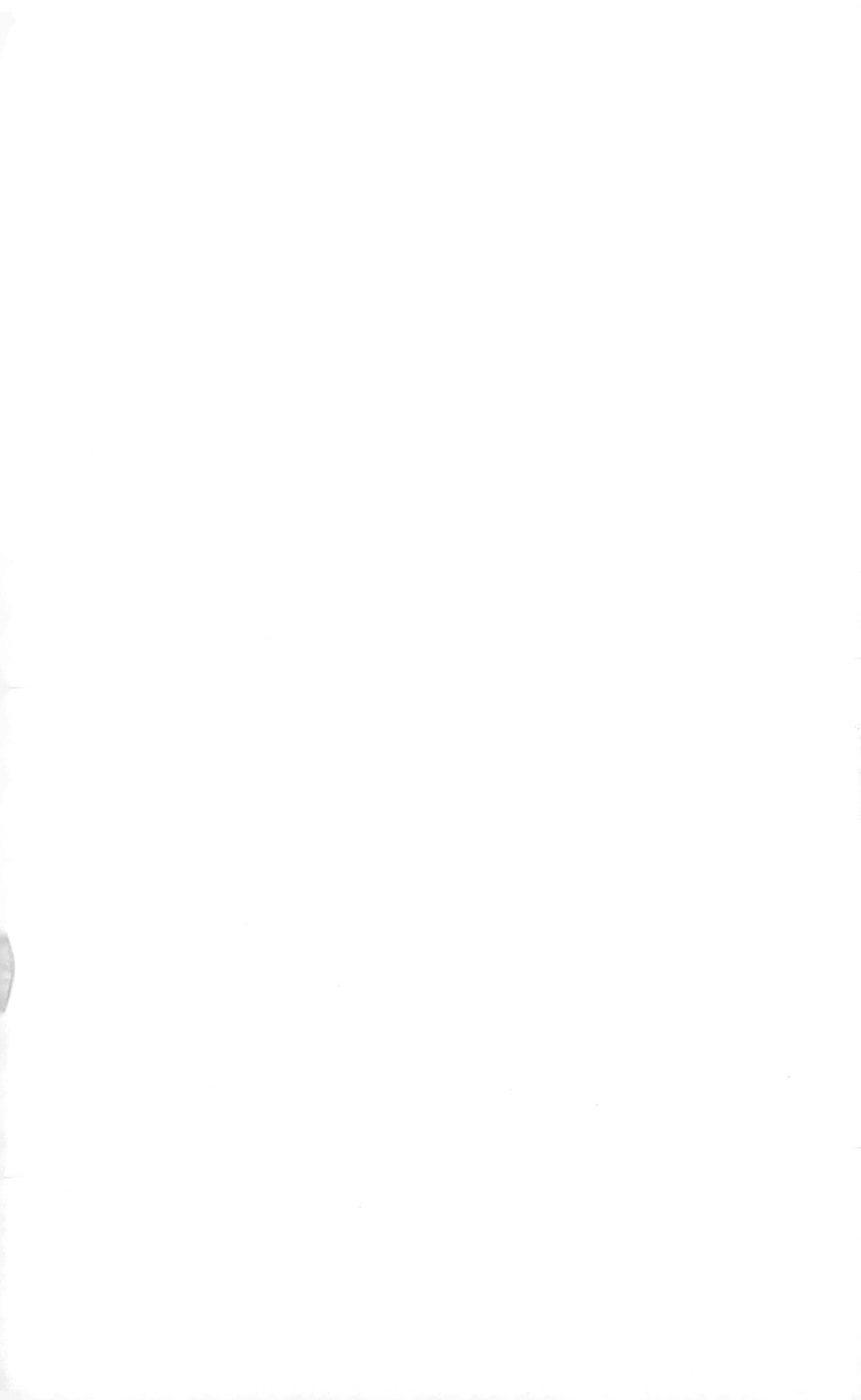